Pharmacology
A Practical Manual
for Medical Students

As per the latest
CBME Guidelines |
Competency Based Undergraduate Curriculum
for the Indian Medical Graduate

Pharmacology
A Practical Manual
for Medical Students

As per the latest
CBME Guidelines |
Competency Based Undergraduate Curriculum
for the Indian Medical Graduate

Rajesh Kumar Suman
Assistant Professor
Department of Pharmacology
Hind Institute of Medical Sciences
Ataria, Sitapur, Lucknow

Ipseeta Ray Mohanty
Professor
Department of Pharmacology
MGM Medical College
Navi Mumbai

Manjusha K Borde
Associate Professor
Department of Pharmacology
YMT Dental College and Hospital
Navi Mumbai

Snigdha Misra
Assistant Professor
Department of Pharmacology
MGM Medical College
Navi Mumbai

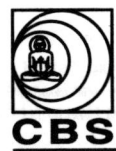

CBS

CBS Publishers & Distributors Pvt Ltd

New Delhi • Bengaluru • Chennai • Kochi • Kolkata • Lucknow • Mumbai
Hyderabad • Jharkhand • Nagpur • Patna • Pune • Uttarakhand

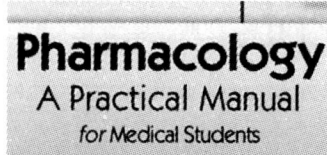

Pharmacology
A Practical Manual
for Medical Students

ISBN: 978-93-90709-88-5

Copyright © Authors and Publisher

First Edition: 2022

Reprint: 2024

Published by Satish Kumar Jain and Produced by Varun Jain for

CBS Publishers & Distributors Pvt Ltd

4819/XI Prahlad Street, 24 Ansari Road, Daryaganj, New Delhi 110 002, India
Ph: 011-23289259, 23266861

Website: www.cbspd.com
e-mail: delhi@cbspd.com

Corporate Office: 204 FIE, Industrial Area, Patparganj, Delhi 110 092
Ph: 011-4934 4934   Fax: 011-4934 4935   e-mail: publishing@cbspd.com; publicity@cbspd.com

Branches

• **Bengaluru:** Seema House 2975, 17th Cross, K.R. Road, Banasankari 2nd Stage, Bengaluru 560 070, Karnataka, India
Ph: +91-80-26771678/79   Fax: +91-80-26771680   e-mail: bangalore@cbspd.com

• **Chennai:** 7, Subbaraya Street, Shenoy Nagar, Chennai 600 030, Tamil Nadu, India
Ph: +91-44-26680620, 26681266   Fax: +91-44-42032115   e-mail: chennai@cbspd.com

• **Kochi:** 42/1325, 1326, Power House Road, Opp KSEB, Power House, Ernakulam 682 018, Kerala, India
Ph: +91-484-4059061-65   Fax: +91-484-4059065   e-mail: kochi@cbspd.com

• **Kolkata:** 147, Hind Ceramics Compound, 1st Floor, Nilgunj Road, Belghoria, Kolkata-700056
West Bengal, India
Ph: 033-25633055, 033-25633056   e-mail: kolkata@cbspd.com

• **Lucknow:** Basement, Khushnuma Complex, 7-Meerabai Marg (Behind Jawahar Bhawan), Lucknow 226001, India
Ph: 0522-4000032   e-mail: tiwari.lucknow@cbspd.com

• **Mumbai:** PWD Shed. Gala no. 25/26, Ramchandra Bhatt Marg, Next to JJ Hospital Gate no. 2, Opp. Union Bank of India Noorbaug
Mumbai-400009, Maharashtra, India
Ph: 022-66661880/89   e-mail: mumbai@cbspd.com

Representatives

• **Hyderabad** 0-9885175004 • **Jharkhand** 0-9811541605 • **Nagpur** 0-8692091830
• **Patna** 0-9334159340 • **Pune** 0-9664372571 • **Uttarakhand** 0-9716462459

Printed at Glorious Printers, Jhilmil Industrial Area, Delhi, India *to*

My Teacher

Late Dr Yeshwant Deshmukh

Former Professor and Head, Department of Pharmacology

MGM Medical College, Navi Mumbai

and

My Parents

Shree Nand Lal Shah and Smt Jyantri Devi Shah

Foreword

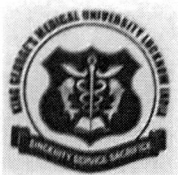

KING GEORGE'S MEDICAL UNIVERSITY, U.P. LUCKNOW
Department of Pharmacology & Therapeutics
Ph.0522-2257448

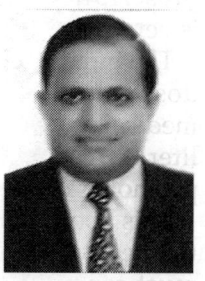

It is indeed a great pleasure for me to write foreward for the book *Pharmacology: A Practical Manual for Medical Students* authored by Dr Rajesh Kumar Suman, et al. which will be published by CBS Publishers & Distributors, New Delhi. The book explains practical aspects under broad chapters like clinical pharmacology, pharmacy, experimental pharmacology and protocol writing. The book covers the content that are essential for medical students like prescription writing, rational drug use, drug dose calculation, drug interaction, adverse drug reaction, new drug development, problem based learning exercises, pharmacy preparations, dosage forms and animal experiments are well explained. The book also covers techniques to administer drug through various routes which will be helpful for skill assessment on mannequins.

Unique feature of this book is concise presentation of protocol writing and information about ICMR-STS project for undergraduate students so students could write protocol for short-term studentship research projects which has been sponsored by ICMR to enhance undergraduate research.

Dr Rajesh Kumar Suman to has taken good effort to present this book in a simple manner and, cover every aspects for practical pharmacology which should be taught in 2nd semester professional MBBS curriculum. I hope, this book will become an essential tool for students as well as teachers to understand practical pharmacology. I deem it privilege to recommend this practical book for pharmacology, which is concise and lucidely presented.

I congratulate and wish all the best to Dr Rajesh

Dr Amod Kumar Sachan
Professor and Head
Department of Pharmacology and Therapeutics
KGMU, Lucknow

Foreword

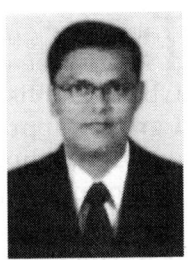

We have ushered in the era of Competency Based Medical Education (CBME). This change in curriculum necessitated the availability of appropriate books and manuals to guide teachers and students alike in this new system. CBME gives more stress on practical aspects and so far as pharmacology is concerned, there is a lot at stake as drugs used by patients is so common place. Starting from the concept of P-drugs to writing a proper prescription and communicating the same effectively to the patient is very important.

The importance of knowledge of various dosage froms, drug delivery systems and dose calculations, etc. therefore can't be overemphasized. We want to train our medical undergraduates on pharmacovigilance, critical appraisal of drug promotional literatures and interaction with medical representatives which ultimately would promote rational drug prescription by these budding doctors.

This book *Pharmacology: A Practical Manual for Medical Students* does a fair justice to the newly introduced curriculum and fills the gap between demand and supply. I must congratulate the authors and editors on taking this painstaking effort towards writing this much needed book. The idea of introducing a chapter on ICMR-STS project is brilliant and contemporary. I am sure that medical students would find this manual very useful not only during their student days but also in future when they become doctors.

Dr Bhabagrahi Rath
Professor and Head
Department of Pharmacology and In-charge Registrar
Formerly In-charge Controller of Examinations
VSS Institute of Medical Sciences and Research (VIMSAR)
Burla, Sambalpur, Odisha-768017
E mail: rathbhabagrahi@gmail.com

Foreword

I am very glad to know that you have written a book entitled *Pharmacology: A Practical Manual for Medical Students* which is being published by CBS Publishers & Distributors, New Delhi. I greatly appreciate the effort taken by you to publish such a wonderful book. Hope, this book will help students a lot in understanding practical aspects of pharmacology in a very easy way.

It is a great accomplishment and my heartiest congratulation to you. Hind Institute of Medical Sciences will extend all possible support in this endeavor.

With best wishes

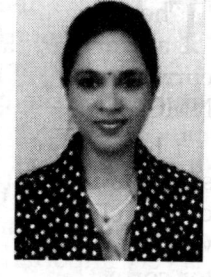

Dr Richa Mishra
Chairperson
Hind Institute of Medical Sciences
Mau, Ataria, Sitapur

Preface

The great developments/advances in pharmacology during the last two decades are accountable for being one of the most important subjects in medical curriculum. This book covers contents as per the new curriculum implemented by NMC.

I have tried to design this book in a simple and presentable form to make students understand the practical aspects of pharmacology. This book elaborately covers clinical pharmacology, pharmacy, experimental pharmacology, protocol writing and communication with patient/representative. Solved exercises are given for correct prescription writing, how to criticise and correct a prescription, adverse drug reaction and drug interaction, etc. to impart problem based learning. The book also covers solved exercises on pharmacy preparations which will facilitate undergraduate research. As ICMR provides stipend to MBBS and BDS students to participate in research, therefore I have included every aspect to write, design and to submit protocol for ICMR-STS projects.

I hope my purposeful attempt will help students and teachers alike in their future endeavor and learning. For any feedback, write to me at rajeshsuman2043@gmail.com.

Rajesh Kumar Suman

Acknowledgement

I wish to sincerely acknowledge all the extremely special people who has done great help to bring this book. I am very much thankful to Dr HK Singh, Professor and Head, Department of Pharmacology, Hind Institute of Medical Sciences, for editing of the book. His inspiring guidance, motivation, enthusiasm, perpetual encouragement, valuable advice and extensive discussions during writing this book have enabled me to successfully complete the task. I am thankful to Dr Savita Sahani, former Professor and Head, Department of Pharmacology, MGM Medical College, for reviewing and providing me valuable suggestion regarding content of this book.

I am grateful to Professors of Pediatrics, Dr NC Mohanty, Ex Medical Superintendent, MGM Hospital, Kalamboli, Navi Mumbai. I had published my first research paper under his umbrella and guidance.

I take the opportunity to convey my heartfelt gratitude to Dr Sanjay Khanna and Dr Tariq Salman, Professor, Department of Pharmacology, HIMS, Sitapur. I extend my sincere thanks to Dr Swapnil Srivastava, Associate Professor; Dr Priti Singh, Assistant Professor; Mr Arun Adhikari, Tutor, and Dr Gulam Mohammad, Tutor, HIMS, Sitapur.

My humble and sincere gratitude are due to Dr Anurag Pathak, Assistant Professor, NIMS, Jaipur, for his support during writing this book.

I thanks to Dr Vithal Patil, Associate Professor, Bharti Vidyapeeth Dental College, Navi Mumbai; Dr Yogesh Garje, Medical Advisor, Sun Pharma, for their support.

My special thanks to Dr Rakesh Kumar, Surgeon (ENT), Lokbandhu Hospital, Lucknow, and my wife Mrs Soni Shah, for her unconditional and emotional support.

No words can describe the feeling of gratitude and admiration for Dr Ipseeta Ray Mohanty, my guide and mentor, without her enthusiastic and acuminous guidance, I would not have been able to complete this book.

I thank Mr SK Jain, CMD and Mr YN Arjuna, Senior Vice President—Publishing, Editorial and Publicity, CBS Publishers & Distributors, New Delhi, for their support.

Rajesh Kumar Suman

Contents

Foreword by Amod Kumar Sachan   vi
Foreword by Bhabagrahi Rath   vii
Foreword by Richa Mishra   viii
Preface   ix
Index of Competencies   xiii

SECTION A: CLINICAL PHARMACOLOGY

1. Prescription Writing   3

2. Relevant Clinical Pharmacokinetic Parameters and Drug Dose Calculation   19

3. Teaching of Rational Drug Use   22

4. Monitoring Adverse Drug Reactions   27

5. Problem Based Exercise on Adverse Drug Reaction   35

6. Identify and Describe the Management of Drug Interactions   41

7. Problem Based Exercise on Drug Interaction   47

8. Critical Appraisal of Drug Promotional Literature   49

9. New Drug Discovery   52

10. Problem Based Learning   57

11. Criticism on Prescription   63

12. Skill Assessment on Mannequin: Administration of Medication by Various Route (DOAP)   71

SECTION B: CLINICAL PHARMACY

13. Introduction to Pharmacy   89

14. Standard Abbreviations   95

15. Route of Drug Administration   96

16. Dosage Forms   104

17. Pharmacy Preparations   113

SECTION C: EXPERIMENTAL PHARMACOLOGY

18. Introduction to Experimental Pharmacology   147

19. Regulations for Use of Animals for Experiments and Research   149

20. Animals Used in Experimental Pharmacology   150

21. Animal Experiments   152

SECTION D: PROTOCOL WRITING

22. Protocol Writing   163

23. How to Write ICMR-STS Project by Under Graduate Students   170

SECTION E: COMMUNICATION SKILL

24. Interaction with Pharmaceutical Representative   177

25. Communication with the Patients   179

Index of Competencies

Practical Competencies Covered	Competency Number	Page No.
Enumerate and identify drug formulations and drug delivery route	PH 1.3	98, 104
Demonstrate understanding of the use of various dosage forms **(oral/local/parenteral; solid/liquid)**	PH 2.1	104
Prepare oral rehydration solution from ORS packet and explain its use	PH 2.2	113, 140
Administer drugs through various routes in a simulated environment using mannequins	PH 4.1	71
Demonstrate the appropriate setting up of an intravenous drip in a simulated environment	PH 2.3	83
Demonstrate the correct method of calculation of drug dosage in patients including those used in special situations	PH 1.12, 2.4	19
Write a rational, correct and legible generic prescription for a given condition and communicate the same to the patient	PH 3.1	3
Describe parts of correct, complete and legible generic prescription. Identify errors in prescription and correct appropriately	PH 1.10	63
Interpret critical appraisal of a given prescription	PH 3.2	49, 63
Perform a critical evaluation of the drug promotional literature	PH 3.3	49
To recognise and report an adverse drug reaction	PH 1.6	27
Define, identify and describe the management of adverse drug reactions	PH 1.7	31
Identify and describe management of drug interaction	PH 1.8	41
To prepare and explain a list of P-drugs for a given case	PH 3.5	25
Essential Medicine concept	PH 3.7	25
Demonstrate the effects of drugs on blood pressure (vasopressor and vasodepressors with appropriate blockers) using CAL	PH 4.2	152
Communication effectively with a patient on the proper use of prescribed medication	PH 3.8	179
Demonstrate how to optimize interaction with pharmaceutical representative to get authentic information on drugs	PH 3.6	177

Clinical Pharmacology

1. Prescription Writing

2. Relevant Clinical Pharmacokinetic Parameters and Drug Dose Calculation

3. Teaching of Rational Drug Use

4. Monitoring Adverse Drug Reactions

5. Problem Based Exercise on Adverse Drug Reaction

6. Identify and Describe the Management of Drug Interactions

7. Problem Based Exercise on Drug Interaction

8. Critical Appraisal of Drug Promotional Literature

9. New Drug Development

10. Problem Based Learning

11. Criticism on Prescription

12. Skill Assessment on Mannequin: Administration of Medication by Various Route (DOAP)

Prescription Writing

INTRODUCTION

The prescription order is an important therapeutic transaction between physician and patients. It brings into focus the diagnostic acumen and therapeutic proficiency of the physician with instruction, for palliation or restoration of the patient's health. It is a written order by a qualified clinician to the pharmacist to dispense medical substances for the patient. It consists the instruction to the pharmacist regarding dispensing of drug, the amount required and also directions of application to the patients.

It is a medicolegal document and hence it should be written with caution. The prescription should not only be accurate and precise, but should be written in a specific pattern with particular care to avoid possibilities of error or misinterpretation on the part of pharmacist/chemist/patient.

Essentials of prescription

1. Selection of drug
2. Selection of the dosage form
3. Knowledge of posology
4. Knowledge of drug combination
5. Knowledge of drug interaction

Parts of prescription:

1. **Superscription:** Includes the following interaction:
    a. Doctors name, Address, Registration No. and Date, the registration number is allotted by regional medical council. It is essential to quote this in all prescription.
    b. Patient name, Age, Sex and Address.
    c. The sign ℞ means Recipe or take thou, this also represents mythologically prayer to Jupiter, 'the God of health'. A symbol, which is to be written on outside left at the top of the body of prescription.

2. **Inscription:** This is also called body of prescription. Inscription differs according to the availability of prescribed medication. A precompounded medication is a drug or a mixture of drug supplied by the pharmaceutical company. A compounded medication is the one prepared by pharmacist according to clinician's order.

When the preparation is a compounded medication the drugs prescribed are written as follows:

    a. Basis: Active drug

    b. Adjuvant: Substance intended to assist and especially hasten the action of the basis.

    c. Corrective: Substances which corrects the undesirable action of basis and or of the adjuvant.

    d. Vehicle or excipient: Substance which carries the above ingredients.

3. **Subscription:** It contains direction to the pharmacist as to the mode of compounding, amount to be compounded the form of the final medicament and division into doses if required.

4. **Transcription:** This consists of direction to the patient regarding the method of administration, the dose (if given orally), the time of administration, any other instruction (label is also called as transcription)

5. **Signature of doctor:** Essential to make the prescription valid.

The following points should be remembered while writing a prescription

1. The writing should be legible. The drug names should be in capital letters so that they are legible.

2. Abbreviations should be avoided.

3. Generic name of drugs should be prefered.

4. If there is more than one dosage form given by different routes, the order should be as follows.

Injection followed by:

- Oral preparations in this order
- Capsules, tablets, liquids and
- Finally topical preparation

Note: It is preferable to write a prescription on the Doctor's own letterhead and the Physician must preserve a copy of the prescription.

Parts of Prescription and Model of Prescription:

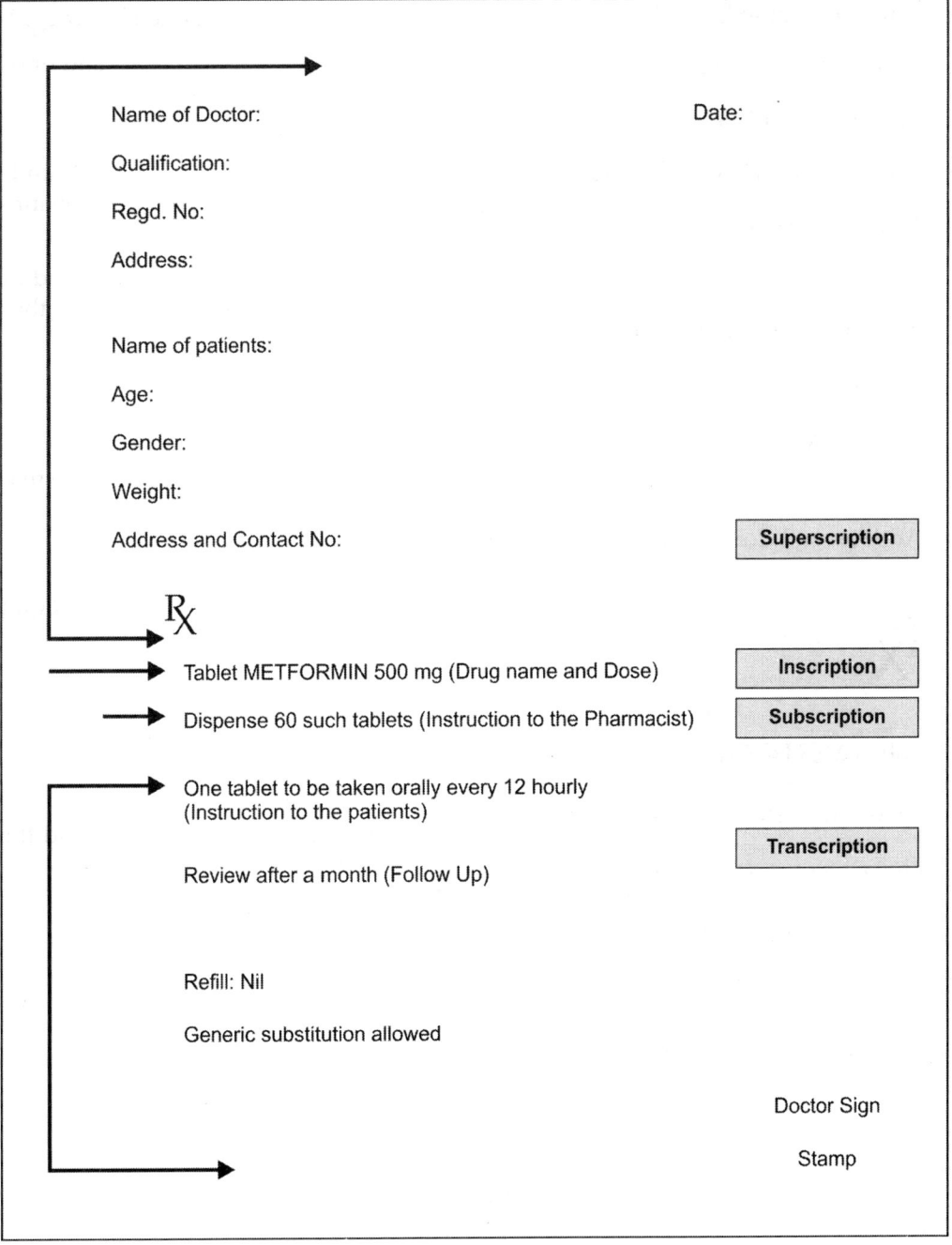

Name of Doctor: Date:

Qualification:

Regd. No:

Address:

Name of patients:

Age:

Gender:

Weight:

Address and Contact No: **Superscription**

℞

Tablet METFORMIN 500 mg (Drug name and Dose)   **Inscription**

Dispense 60 such tablets (Instruction to the Pharmacist)   **Subscription**

One tablet to be taken orally every 12 hourly
(Instruction to the patients)

                                                       Transcription

Review after a month (Follow Up)

Refill: Nil

Generic substitution allowed

                                        Doctor Sign

                                        Stamp

Fig. 1.1

1. Prescribe drug therapy for 40 year old male who is suffering from type 2 diabetes mellitus.

Name of Doctor: Dr ABC   Date 11/12/2020

MBBS, MD (Medicine)

Regd No: MCI 123

Address: Indra Nagar, Lucknow

Mob no: 123456

Name of patients: Mr. Kumar

Age: 40 year

Gender: Male

Weight: 70 kg

Address and Contact No: Ataria, Sitapur

R$_X$

Tablet METFORMIN 500 mg

Dispense 60 such tablets

One tablet to be taken orally every 12 hourly

Review after a month

Refil: Nil

Generic substitution allowed   Doctor Sign

                                                   Stamp

Fig. 1.2

2. Prescribe drug therapy for 40 year old male who has been diagnosed with epilepsy.

Name of Doctor: Dr ABC   Date 11/12/2020

MBBS, MD (Medicine)

Regd No: MCI 123

Address: Indra Nagar, Lucknow

Mob no: 123456

Name of patients: Mr. Kumar

Age: 40 year

Gender: Male

Weight: 70 kg

Address and Contact No.: Ataria, Sitapur

Tablet PHENYTOIN   100 mg

Dispense 90 such tablets

One tablet to be taken orally every 8 hourly

Review after a month

Refil: Nil

Generic substitution allowed   Doctor Sign

                                                          Stamp

---

Fig. 1.3

3. Prescribe drug for 40 year old female diagnosed with typhoid fever.

Name of Doctor: Dr ABC   Date 10/12/2020

MBBS, MD (Medicine)

Regd No: MCI 123

Address: Indra Nagar, Lucknow

Mob no: 123456

Name of patients: Mrs. Rohini

Age: 40 year

Gender: Female

Weight: 70 kg

Address and Contact No.: Ataria, Sitapur

R̺x

Tablet CIPROFLOXACIN   750 mg

Dispense 20 such tablets

One tablet to be taken orally every 12 hourly

Tablet PARACETAMOL   500 mg

Dispense 20 such tablets

One tablet to be taken orally every 6 hourly (if fever)

Review after 10 days

Refil: Nil

Generic substitution allowed   Doctor Sign

                                                          Stamp

---

Fig. 1.4

4. Prescribe drug therapy for 52 year old male patient diagnosed with tuberculosis.

Name of Doctor: Dr ABC   Date 09/11/2020

MBBS, MD (Medicine)

Regd No: MCI 123

Address: Indra Nagar, Lucknow

Mob no: 123456

Name of patients: Mr. Kumar

Age: 52 year

Gender: Male

Weight: 70 kg

Address and Contact No.: Ataria, Sitapur

Rχ

Tablet ISONIAZID   300 mg

Dispense 60 such tablets

One tablet to be taken orally every 24 hourly

Tablet RIFAMPICIN   600 mg

Dispense 60 such tablets

One tablet to be taken orally every 24 hourly on empty stomach

Tablet PYRAZINAMIDE   1 gm

Dispense   60 such tablets

One tablet to be taken orally every 24 hourly

Tablet ETHAMBUTOL   1 gm

Dispense 60 such tablets

One tablet to be taken orally every 24 hourly

Review after 2 months

Refil: Nil

Generic substitution allowed   Doctor Sign

                                   Stamp

Fig. 1.5

5. Prescribe drug therapy for 40 year old male with status asthmaticus.

Name of Doctor: Dr ABC   Date 05/12/2020

MBBS, MD (Medicine)

Regd No: MCI 123

Address: Indra Nagar, Lucknow

Mob no: 123456

Name of patients: Mr. Kumar

Age: 40 year

Gender: Male

Weight: 70 kg

Address and contact No.: Ataria. Sitapur

Injection HYDROCORTISONE HEMISUCCINATE 100 mg per vial

Dispense 1 such vial

One injection to be taken intravenously stat

Respiratory solution SALBUTAMOL 2.5 mg per 5 ml

Dispense 4 such neubules

One neubule to be aerolized stat

Respiratory solution IPRATROPIUM BROMIDE 0.5 mg per 2.5 ml

Dispense 4 such neubules

One neubule to be aerolized stat

HUMIDIFIED OXYGEN

Administer at a rate of 6-8 lit/min

Review every 4 hour

Refil: Nil

Generic substitution allowed

Doctor sign

Stamp

Fig. 1.6

6. Prescribe drug therapy for 40 year old female suffering from peptic ulcer.

Name of Doctor: Dr ABC

MBBS, MD (Medicine)

Regd No: MCI 123

Address: Indra Nagar, Lucknow

Mob no: 123456

Name of patients: Mr Geeta

Age: 40 year

Gender: Female

Weight: 60 kg

Address and contact No.: Ataria, Sitapur

Capsule LANSOPRAZOLE 30 mg

Dispense 14 such capsule

One capsule to be taken orally every 24 hourly on empty stomach

Capsule AMOXYCILLIN 500 mg

Dispense 56 such capsule

Two capsule to be taken orally every 12 hourly

Tablet CLARITHROMYCIN 500 mg

Dispense 28 such tablets

One tablet to be taken orally every 12 hourly

Review after 2 week

Refil: Nil

Generic substitution allowed   Doctor sign

                                         Stamp

Fig. 1.7

7. Prescribe drug therapy for 50 year old male patients with newly diagnosed mild hypertension.

Name of Doctor: Dr ABC

MBBS, MD (Medicine)

Regd No: MCI 123

Address: Indra Nagar, Lucknow

Mob no: 123456

Name of patients: Mr Kumar

Age: 50 year

Gender: Male

Weight: 70 kg

Address and contact No.: Ataria, Sitapur

R̶X

Tablet ENALAPRIL 2.5 mg

Dispense 30 such tablets

One tablet to be taken orally every 24 hourly

Review after 1 month

Refil: Nil

Generic substitution allowed

Doctor sign

Stamp

Fig. 1.8

8. Prescribe drug therapy for 55 year old male with acute angina pectoris.

Name of Doctor: Dr ABC   Date: 12/12/2020

MBBS, MD (Medicine)

Regd No: MCI 123

Address: Indra Nagar, Lucknow

Mob no: 123456

Name of patients: Mr. Kumar

Age: 55 year

Gender: Male

Weight: 70 kg

Address and contact No.: Ataria, Sitapur

Tablet GLYCERYLTRINITRATE   0.6 mg

Dispense 3 such tablets

One tablet to be taken sublingually stat

Repeat every 5 min till symptoms subside (maximum 3 time can be used)

Review after sometime

Refil: Nil

Generic substitution allowed   Doctor sign

                                                        Stamp

---

Fig. 1.9

9. Prescribe drug therapy for 50 year old female diagnosed with hypothyroidism.

Name of Doctor: Dr ABC

MBBS, MD (Medicine)

Regd No: MCI 123

Address: Indra Nagar, Lucknow

Mob no: 123456

Name of patients: Mrs. Site

Age: 50 year

Gender: Female

Weight: 70 kg

Address and contact No.: Ataria, Sitapur

R̥x

Tablet LEVOTHYROXINE   50 mg

Dispense 30 such tablets

One tablet to be taken orally every 24 hourly on empty stomach

Review after 1 month

Refil: Nil

Generic substitution allowed   Doctor sign

                                                                              Stamp

---

Fig. 1.10

10. Prescribe drug therapy for 35 year old female diagnosed with *P. vivax* malaria.

Name of Doctor: Dr ABC   Date: 10/12/2020

MBBS, MD (Medicine)

Regd No: MCI 123

Address: Indra Nagar, Lucknow

Mob no: 123456

Name of patients: Mrs. Sita

Age: 35 year

Gender: Female

Weight: 70 kg

Address and contact No.: Ataria, Sitapur

Tablet CHLOROQUINE   600 mg, 300 mg

Dispense 1 (600 mg) such tablets

Dispense 3 (300 mg) such tablets

One tablet (600 mg) to be taken orally stat and after 6 hours one tablet (300 mg) to be taken orally and one tab on 2nd and 3rd day

Tablet PRIMAQUINE 15 mg

Dispense 10 such tablets

One tablet to be taken orally every 24 hourly from day 4 to day 14

Review after a week

Refil: Nil

Generic substitution allowed   Doctor sign

                                                         Stamp

---

Fig. 1.11

11. Prescribe drug therapy for 24 year old male suffering with motion sickness.

Name of Doctor: Dr ABC   Date: 05/11/2020

MBBS, MD (Medicine)

Regd No: MCI 123

Address: Indra Nagar, Lucknow

Mob no: 123456

Name of patients: Mr Bikash

Age: 24 year

Gender: Male

Weight: 70 kg

Address and contact No.: Ataria, Sitapur

℞

Tablet PROMETHAZINE   50 mg

Dispense 2 such tablets

One tablet to be taken orally one hour before starting journey

Review after a day

Refil: Nil

Generic substitution allowed   Doctor sign

                                                          Stamp

---

Fig. 1.12

12. Prescribe drug therapy for anaphylactic reaction.

Name of Doctor: Dr ABC　　　　　　　　　　　　　Date: 11/12/2020

MBBS, MD (Medicine)

Regd No: MCI 123

Address: Indra Nagar, Lucknow

Mob no: 123456

Name of patients: Mr Vivek

Age: 40 year

Gender: Male

Weight: 70 kg

Address and contact No.: Ataria, Sitapur

Injection ADRENALINE 0.5 ml (1:1000)

Dispense 1 such prefilled syrings

Inject 0.5 ml intramuscularly stat

Injection HYDROCORTISONE HEMISUCCINATE 100 mg, 500 mg

Dispense such 1 vial of 100 mg and 1 vial of 500 mg

Inject 100 mg intravenously stat and 500 mg via intravenous drip

Injection DOPAMINE HCL 40 mg

Dispense such 1 vial of 5 ml

5 ml dissolved in 250 ml of normal saline and infused at the rate of 5 mg/kg/min

Refil: Nil

Generic substitution allowed　　　　　　　　　　　Doctor sign

　　　　　　　　　　　　　　　　　　　　　　　　　　Stamp

Fig. 1.13

13. Prescribe drug therapy for 40 year male with acute attack of migraine.

Name of Doctor: Dr ABC   Date: 11/12/2020

MBBS, MD (Medicine)

Regd No: MCI 123

Address: Indra Nagar, Lucknow

Mob no: 123456

Name of patients: Mr. Vivek

Age: 40 year

Gender: Male

Weight: 70 kg

Address and contact No.: Ataria, Sitapur

℞

Tablet SUMATRIPTAN 50 mg

Dispense 4 such tablets

One tablet to be taken orally. If attack do not subside, repeat after 2 hours upto a total dose of 200 mg over a period of 24 hours

Review after a day

Refil: Nil

Generic substitution allowed   Doctor sign

                                          Stamp

Fig. 1.14

Relevant Clinical Pharmacokinetic Parameters and Drug Dose Calculation

Clearance: Volume of plasma from which a drug is cleared/removed in unit time and expressed in ml/min.

Example: Clearance of a drug 500 ml/min, means 500 ml of plasma is cleared of that particular drug.

$$CL = \text{Rate of elimination/plasma concentration}$$

Creatinine clearance: Renal clearance is measured by GFR, creatinine clearance can be calculated from serum creatinine value using formula of Cockcroft and Gault.

$$\text{Creatinine clearance} = (140 - \text{age}) \times (\text{weight in kg})/72 \times \text{serum creatinine (for male)}$$

For female, the value can be multiplied by 0.85.

Steady state concentration: If drug is administered at a constant rate, the plasma concentration of drug rises and state is achieved at which the rate of administration (dose rate) of drug is exactly equal to rate of elimination is called *steady state concentration* (SSC).

$$SSC = \text{Dose rate/CL}$$

Maintenance dose: After, loading dose, the amount of drug eliminated daily is usually, the administered daily and is called *maintenance dose* (MD), i.e. to maintain the therapeutic plasma concentration achieved. MD is smaller and sometime 1/4th of loading dose.

$$\text{Dose rate IV} = \text{Rate of elimination at SSC} = mg/h$$

$$= CL/(L/h) \times \text{therapeutic plasma concentration (TPC)}$$

$$\text{Dose rate (oral)} = \text{Dose rate/bioavailability (F)}$$

$$\text{Oral MD} = \text{Dose rate (amount/h)} \times \text{dosing interval (h)/F oral}$$

$$= CL \times TPC \times \text{dosing interval (h)/F oral}$$

$$= \text{Amount/kg/h}$$

Revised Dose

Steady state concentration in patients depends on F, Vd and CL and there is significant variation from patients to patients in these parameters. Measurement of plasma concentration enables to adjust the dose in a patient. Considering that the drug follows first order kinetics (for most of the drug), the revised dose can be calculated as follows:

Revised dose = Previous dose × required target plasma concentration/measured plasma concentration

DOSE CALCULATIONS
Dose Calculation on the Basis of Age

1. **Young's formula:** It is presumed that a 12 years old child should be given half of the adult dose

$$\text{Child's dose} = \text{Age in years}/\text{age} +12 \times \text{adult dose}$$

   Example: Adult dose of paracetamol is 500 mg, calculate for child dose?
$$\text{Child's dose} = 12/12 + 12 \times 500$$
$$= 250 \text{ mg}$$

2. **Dilling's formula:** It is presumed that 20 years old adult should be given adult dose

$$\text{Child's dose} = \text{Age in years}/20 \times \text{adult dose}$$

   Example:
   Calculate the dose of paracetamol for 20 years old
$$\text{Child's dose} = 20/20 \times 500$$
$$= 500 \text{ mg}$$

Dose calculation on the basis of weight (Clark's formula): It is simply based on presumption that adult weight is 70 kg or 150 lbs and thus accordingly dose of a child can be calculated based on per kg body weight.

a. Child dose = Weight of child in kg/70 × adult dose
b. Child dose = Weight of child in pounds (lbs)/150 × adult dose

Example: Calculate the dose of paracetamol for 20 kg child
$$\text{Child' dose} = 20/70 \times 500$$
$$= 142.85 \text{ mg}$$

Dose calculation on the basis of body surface area: The body surface area (BSA) is a better index because it is based on both the height and weight. Moreover, metabolism including drug metabolism is also related with BSA. Thus, BSA is precise, better and more accurate index to calculate dose in a child, however, it may not be of much important in adults (Dubois formula).

$$\text{Child's dose} = \text{BSA (m}^2)/1.73 \times \text{adult dose}$$

BSA of an individual can be calculated as follows:

$$\text{BSA (m}^2) = \text{BW (kg)}^{0.425} \times \text{height (cm)}^{0.725} \times 0.007184$$

Average adult body weight: The dose can also be calculated by using the average adult body weight (60–70 kg) basis from the formula:

$$\text{Individual dose} = \text{Body weight (kg)}/70 \times \text{average adult dose}$$

Dose Calculation on Renal Dysfunction

Renal disease alters the effects of many drugs, sometimes decreasing their effects but more often increasing their effects and thus potential toxicity. Many of these changes are predictable and can be mitigated by changing drug doses.

Estimates of glomerular filtration rate (GFR) are used to determine renal function, in diagnosing renal disease and are also used to estimate renal drug clearance. Some active drug moieties are wholly or partly cleared from the body by the kidneys and this is the physiological rationale for using GFR to estimate drug clearance.

The units of drug dose are amount per unit time, e.g. 500 mg twice daily. For most drugs, prescribing information recommends a standard dose and provides some guidance on when this should be changed. The advice is necessarily imprecise as most drugs have large inter-individual variability in clearance and response. Consequently, dose adjustment is crude for most drugs in most circumstances, for example by doubling or halving doses. This is reflected in the available drug preparations, with most provided in a limited number of strengths which limits dose adjustment options. In most case having a means to identify when drug dose should be halved or doubled is important, whereas a 20% change in dose is usually impractical or unnecessary. However, there are several drugs for which small changes in dose or concentration may have an important effect, commonly known as a *narrow therapeutic index*.

For drugs with narrow therapeutic indices, a small change in drug concentration can cause toxicity or loss of efficacy. Narrow therapeutic index drugs should be dosed using robust biomarkers, as estimates or empirical calculations of dose are not reliable enough to be safe. For example, lithium is a renally cleared drug with a narrow therapeutic index; therapeutic drug monitoring is used together with clinical response to guide dosing. Warfarin is a narrow therapeutic index drug that is metabolized rather than renally cleared; international normalized ratio (INR) is used as a biomarker to guide dosing.

Drug Clearance

Drug clearance (CL) and bioavailability (F) (the fraction of the drug dose that reaches the systemic circulation) determine the steady state plasma concentration (Cp) at a given dose. CL has the units of volume/time and F is dimensionless (%). Note that CL is not the same as drug elimination (which like dose has units of amount/time and becomes equal to dose at steady state).

$$\text{Dose} = \text{Cp} \times \text{CL/F mg/h or mg/L} \tag{1}$$

Cp = Steady state plasma concentration
CL = Drug clearance
 F = Bioavailability

From Eq (1), it can be seen that if CL is halved, drug dose should be halved to keep the drug concentration the same. Thus, if a drug is 100% renally cleared and renal function is half-normal, the drug dose should be halved, all other variables being equal. However, many drugs are inactivated by metabolism (in the liver predominantly), and hence doses of metabolized drugs do not usually require changing in renal disease.

Teaching of Rational Drug Use

Rational drug use is conventionally defined as " the use of an appropriate, efficacious, safe and cost-effective drug given for the right indication in the right dose and formulation, at right intervals and for the right duration of time." Irrational use of medications results in inadequate and dangerous treatment, leading to aggravation or prolongation of disease and adverse effects of the drug. Certainly, examples of useless, ineffective and unacceptable drugs should be clearly and explicitly quoted, and physicians taught to recognize their like when they encounter them in practice; this will assist the future prescriber to appreciate the difference between trying to manage clinical problems and merely looking for drug indications. Beyond that, however, teaching must concentrate on essentials: Clinical and epidemiological problems and challenges. If one is to teach the therapeutic strategies needed to approach common and dominant clinical problems, an undergraduate teaching programme in clinical pharmacology should cover some key areas that are not handled by other clinical disciplines. These will include reading and interpreting clinical trial reports, understanding the potential therapeutic implications of pharmacokinetic profiles, appreciating the mechanisms, frequency, severity and diagnosis of the undesirable effects of drugs, and knowing something of the legislative, economic and social aspects of the use of medicines.

One must, however, also pause briefly to consider the development and teaching of clinical pharmacology itself as a specialty in medicine; increasingly it has been realized that such specialists are needed to support the rational use of drugs in society. Prescribing is a complex and challenging task which must be based on accurate and objective information and not an automated action, without critical thinking or a response to commercial pressure. There are worldwide evidences of poor prescribing due to errors, polypharmacy, and inappropriate or irrational prescribing. When medicines are prescribed or used erroneously, they pose serious health risks to the patient and significant associated economic implications

Factors responsible for poor prescribing have been identified, such as deficiency of training, failure to perceive the importance of the task, lack of identifying the errors, and increasing therapeutic options. To overcome these difficulties, the World Health Organization produced the 'Guide to Good Prescribing' which takes the medical student through a structured problem-solved six-step process in choosing and prescribing a suitable drug for an individual patient. The WHO's guide is based on the concept of 'Rational Use of Medicines' (RUM) which requires patients to receive appropriate medications for their clinical needs, in proper individual doses for the correct period of time at a low cost for them and the community.

In prescribing a treatment, the doctor can choose between drug therapy, a combination of drug and non-drug therapy or only a non-drug approach. In the case of a drug based therapy using RUM is essential since it is a process that involves decisions made based on the efficacy, safety, convenience and cost. Furthermore, the correct prescription with the guarantee of access to the prescribed medication and adequate dispensing followed by the proper use by the patient is also part of the RUM principal.

Polypharmacy

The prescription, administration or use of more medication than are clinically indicated in a given patient is called as *polypharmacy*.

Despite the common use of the word 'polypharmacy' for more than 150 years in medical literature, there is no clearly accepted definition. In the past, it was considered poor practice and frowned on to prescribe several medications at the same time to a patient. Increasingly it is recognised that polypharmacy is a 'necessary evil' that for many patients is required to improve clinical outcome. However, it still remains the case that some people are prescribed multiple medications potentially unnecessarily, when they are unlikely to benefit or where drug interactions are likely to cause harm. For these reasons, a definition of polypharmacy where it can be considered either appropriate or problematic is desirable. Furthermore, the use of simple thresholds to define polypharmacy may be unhelpful, and less crude methods are recommended. Polypharmacy is certainly a common and growing global issue, affecting primary and secondary healthcare fundamentals. This is driven by our ageing population and by the increasing levels of multi-morbidity. Numerous evidence-based guidelines help drive the increase in polypharmacy, yet rarely advice on how to manage multi-morbidity. There is a need to have research and guidance that covers commonly associated co-morbidity together with the associated polypharmacy. It is also necessary to address the increasing specialization of clinicians, and the need to train clinicians with specific expertise in managing co-morbidity and clinical complexity, in addition to wider generalist skills. This all requires a significant change in policy and poses a considerable challenge. Further research is also required to examine systems and processes designed to improve medicines management in relation to polypharmacy. Finally, another important challenge in the area of polypharmacy is that of working alongside patients to empower them to make informed choices about treatments and the burden of pills they are expected to consume. Increasingly, it is recognized that many people find their medication regimens an unpleasant chore and this can in its own right detract from their quality of life. If this is not managed well, medicines will not be taken as the prescriber intends, resulting in significant and costly waste, and of course a failure to realise the anticipated benefits of treatment.

Role of doctor to reduce polypharmacy

The medication appropriateness index (MAI) was designed to assist clinicians in assessing the appropriateness of a medication for a given patient. The MAI requires clinicians to rate 10 explicit criteria to determine whether a given medication is appropriate for an individual. For each criterion, the index has operational definitions, explicit instructions and examples alongwith evaluator rates about whether the particular medication is 'appropriate', 'marginally appropriate', or 'inappropriate'.

The 10 explicit criteria are:

i. **Indication:** The sign, symptom, disease or condition for which the medication is prescribed.

ii. **Effectiveness:** Producing a beneficial result.

iii. **Dosage:** Total amount of medication taken per 24 hour period.

iv. **Direction:** Instructions to the patient for the proper use of a medication.

v. **Practicality:** Capability of being used or being put into practice.

vi. **Drug-drug interaction:** The effect that the administration of one medication has on another drug; clinical significance connotes a harmful interaction.

vii. **Drug-disease interaction:** The effect that the drug has on a pre-existing disease or condition; clinical significance connotes a harmful interaction.

viii. **Unnecessary duplication:** Non-beneficial or risky prescribing of two or more drugs from the same chemical or pharmacological class.

ix. **Duration:** Length of therapy.

x. **Expensiveness:** Cost of drug in comparison to other agents of equal efficacy and safety.

Practical Tips on Management of Polypharmacy

1. Never assume your patient is taking what you think they are taking. Regular review is essential. Brown bag reviews (ask the patient to bring all the medicines they are taking to the clinic) or reviews in the patient's home can be illuminating.

2. Keep medication regimens as simple as possible—ideally with once or twice daily dosages. The number of pills or 'pill burden' should be kept to the minimum necessary to provide effective treatment.

3. Provide clear written instructions and a dosing schedule.

4. Ensure that the directions on each prescription item identify the problem it is intended to treat. Be aware of the known pitfalls with specific drugs and recognised drug interactions. You should carefully consider and avoid hazardous prescribing wherever possible.

5. It is important to put systems in place to ensure consistent and appropriate biochemical monitoring takes place for high-risk medicines, e.g. lithium, disease-modifying anti-rheumatic drugs (DMARDs), warfarin.

6. Consider the use of compliance aids such as monitored dosage boxes or 'pill organisers' to improve medicine-taking but be aware that they can also have disadvantages.

7. Discuss complex repeat medication regimens with clinical pharmacy colleagues (both in the community and hospital setting). They can advise on safety, check for hazardous interactions, guide on formulations appropriate to the patient's needs and help in checking patient understanding.

8. Try to ensure that quantities of medication are synchronised so that patients can order their repeat items at the same time and thus avoid potential missed doses and waste.

9. Avoid use of the term 'as directed' and put specific dosage instructions on prescriptions.

10. Always ask your patient if they are using home remedies, such as herbal products or over-the-counter products. Also, could the patient be using somebody else's treatment?

11. Try to substitute rather than add to medication regimens.

12. Think of introducing drugs as a trial: do not forget to stop treatment that is unnecessary or ineffective.

Essential Medicines Concept

WHO has defined; essential medicines are those that satisfy the healthcare needs of majority of the population. They should be of assured quality, available at all times in adequate quantities and in appropriate dosage forms. They should be selected with regards to disease. The original list has undergone revisions and updating from time to time to meet the changing requirements.

WHO has laid down criteria to guide selection of essential drugs

1. Adequate data on its efficacy and safety should be available from clinical studies.

2. Good dosage form ensuring proper bioavailability, stability and quality should be available.

3. It's choice should depends upon pattern of prevalent diseases.

4. In case of two or more similar drugs, choice should be made based on their relative efficacy, safety, quality, price and availability. Cost benefits ratio should be a major consideration.

5. Fixed dose combinations are acceptable only when the dosage of each ingredients meet the requirements of a define population group and the combination has advantage over single drug in therapeutic effects.

6. Selection of essential drugs should be a continue process.

WHO or governments of the country (e.g. governments of India for India) have to prepare the drug list, which contains the names of such essential drugs that is required for most of the people of the country for most of the time. The government of India has published its national essential drugs list in 1996. Only 279 drugs have been included in this. The list was subsequently revised in 2003 with 354 drugs, in 2011 with 348 drugs. The national list of essential medicine was revised in 2015 and contains 376 drugs. A particular drug may be essential in a particular country but need not be so in every country. Thus, snake bite is common in India and antisnake is officially an essential drug in India but need not be so in New Zealand which is officially a snake free country.

P-Drug Concept

P-drugs means preferred or personal drug. P-drugs chosen by a practitioner are essentially the 'drugs of choice' for common conditions, according to his/her own judgment and interpretation. P-drugs will differ from country to country, and between doctors, because of varying availability and cost of drugs, different national formularies and essential drugs lists, medical culture and individual interpretation of information.

A P-drug is selected depending upon the following criteria: Safety: Possible adverse effects. Tolerability: Suitability for a patient. Efficacy: Drug profile. Price: Always look at the total cost of treatment rather than the cost per unit.

For example, nitroglycerine and isosorbide dinitrate sublingual tablets are considered as the P-drugs for the treatment of angina pectoris as compared to other drugs.

Procedure of Choosing a New P-drug

The selection of P-drug is a stepwise process, and the following points should be taken into consideration.

a. Establish a diagnosis
b. Specify the therapeutic objective
c. List the groups of drugs effective in achieving the objective
d. Choose a suitable drug group according to criteria
e. Choose the P-drug

Monitoring Adverse Drug Reactions

ADVERSE DRUG REACTION (ADR)

WHO defined ADR as a noxious, unintended, undesired effect of a drug which occurs at a dose used in man for prophylaxis, treatment or diagnosis of a disease or for modification of physiological state, which compels reduction of dose of the drug or drug withdrawal.

Pharmacovigilance deals with the epidemiologic study of adverse drug effects. It is the science and activities relating to the detection, assessment, understanding and prevention of ADR or other drug/Vaccine related problem.

Adverse event

Any untoward experience encountered by an individual's during the course of clinical trial, which may or may not be associated with drug.

Side effects

Any unintended effects occur at normal dose of the drug, is related to the pharmacological properties of the drug.

Serious adverse event

Any adverse event which is fatal, life threatening, results persistent/ significant disability which results inpatient hospitalization.

Toxicity

It is direct action of the drug usually with high dose of the drug causes damaging the cells.

Dechallenge

This refers to the stopping of the drug, usually after an adverse event (AE) or at the end of a planned treatment. Dechallenge may be complete or partial. That is, the drug is fully stopped or decreased in dose and the AE may fully disappear or only partially decrease.

Rechallenge

This refers to the restarting of the same drug after having stopped it.

Why ADR Monitoring is Essential?

Statistical analysis regarding drug-induced illness revealed:

- ADR causes 2–3% of consultation in general practice
- ADR accounts for 5% of all hospital admissions
- Overall incidence of ADR in hospital in patient departments is 10–20%.

Suspected Adverse Drug Reactions (ADRs) Which Needs to be Reported

1. **Serious adverse event:**
   a. Fatal (e.g. anaphylaxis, ventricular fibrillation)
   b. Life threatening (e.g. torsades de pointes, intracranial bleeding)
   c. Disabling (e.g. optic atrophy)
   d. Incapacitating (e.g. jaundice)
   e. Causing/prolonging hospitalization (e.g. Stevens-Johnson syndrome)

2. **Unexpected adverse event:** Adverse drug experience that has not been adequately observed earlier.

3. **Known adverse reactions (moderate to severe)**
   a. Moderate defined as those reactions requiring dose modification, drug withdrawal, corrective therapy or otherwise significantly affecting the quality of life.
   b. Serious defined as above

4. **Adverse experience relating to:**
   a. New chemical entity
   b. New indications of existing products
   c. New formulations
   d. Novel drug delivery systems
   e. New combinations

5. ADRs in special field of interest such as drug abuse and drug in pregnancy and during lactation.

6. ADRs occurring from overdose or medication error.

7. Unusual lack of efficacy.

Ministry of Health and Family Welfare, Government of India, launched a nationwide Pharmacovigilance programme of India (PVPI) to monitor the safety of medicines in Indian population. Indian Pharmacopoeia commission (IPC) in functioning as National Coordination Centre (NCC) to collate ADR reports and recommend Central Drug Standard Control Organisation (CDSCO) for regulatory intervention.

Who Can Report?

All healthcare professionals (clinicians, dentists, pharmacists, nurses and consumers, etc.) can report ADRs

Why to Report?

As a healthcare professional it is a moral responsibility to report adverse reactions associated with pharmaceutical products to safeguard public health.

What to Report?

PVPI encourages reporting of all types of suspected adverse reactions with all pharmaceutical products irrespective of whether they are known or unknown, serious or non-serious and frequent or rare.

How and Whom to Report?

- A reporter who is not a part of ADR monitoring centres (AMCs) can fill the 'suspected adverse drug reaction reporting form' and can send to the nearest AMC or directly to the NCC
- Or can directly mail the form to pvpi@ipcindia.net or pvpi.ipcindia@gmail.com
- Or can also call on helpline number: 1800-180-3024 to report ADR. ADR reporting form and contact details of AMCs can be downloaded from the official website www.ipc.gov.in

What will Happen to Reported Adverse Drug Reaction form?

The information obtained from your reported ADR form will be entered into the national adverse drug reaction safety database and will be analysed by expert reviewers. This will be helpful in identifying and reducing the risks associated with drugs thus, promotes the safe use of medicines.

Will Reporting have any Negative Consequences on the Healthcare Professionals or the Patient?

- Submission of an ADR report does not have any legal implication on the reporter
- Confidentiality of the reporter and patient will be maintained
- The information is only meant for better understanding of medicines used in India and to safeguard the health of Indian population.

Benefits

1. Generation of drug safety data based on Indian population.
2. Evidence based regulatory decisions can be taken.
3. Educational initiatives to healthcare professionals for improving safe use of medicines.
4. Benefit risk ratio can be assessed.
5. Updation on patient information leaflet-new ADRs, new warnings, new contraindications, dose alteration, etc.
6. Population safety data can be generated-paediatrics, geriatric, pregnancy and lactation.
7. Rational and safe use of medicines can be achieved.
8. Public confidence can be enhanced.

SUSPECTED ADVERSE DRUG REACTION REPORTING FORM

For VOLUNTARY reporting of Adverse Drug Reaction by healthcare professionals

INDIAN PHARMACOPOEIA COMMISSION (National Coordination Centre: Pharmacovigilance programme of India) Ministry of Health & Family Welfare Government of India Sector-23, Raj Nagar, Ghaziabad-201002 www.ipc.nic.in	**(AMC/NCC use only)** AMC Report No. Unique worldwide identification

A. Patient information

1. Patient Initials _____	2. Age at time of event or date of birth _____	3. Sex ☐ M ☐ F 4. Weight _____ kg

B. Patient information

5. Date of reaction started (dd/mm/yyyy)

6. Date of recovery (dd/mm/yyyy)

7. Describe reaction or problem

12. Relevant tests/laboratory data with dates

13. Other relevant history including pre-existing medical conditions (e.g. allergies, race, pregnancy, smoking, alcohol use, hepatic/renal dysfunction, etc.)

14. Seriousness of the reaction

☐ Death (dd/mm/yyyy)   ☐ Congenital-anomaly
☐ Life threatening   ☐ Required intervention to
☐ Hospitalization/prolonged   prevent permanent
☐ Disability   impairment/damage
                            ☐ Other (specify)

15. Outcomes

☐ Fatal   ☐ Recovering   ☐ Unknown
☐ Continuing   ☐ Recovered   ☐ Other (specify)

C. Suspected Medication(s)

S. No.	8. Name (brand and /or generic name)	Manu-facturer (if known)	Batch No./Lot No. (if known)	Exp. Date (if known)	Dose used	Route used	Frequency	Therapy dates (if known, give duration) Date started Date stopped	Reason for use or prescribed for
I.									
II.									
III.									
IV.									

S. No. as per C	9. Reaction abated after drug stopped or dose reduced					10. Reaction reappeared after reintroduction				
	Yes	No	Unknown	NA	Reduced dose	Yes	No	Unknown	NA	If reintroduced, dose
I.										
II.										
III.										
IV.										

11. Concomitant medical product including self-medication and herbal remedies with therapy dates (exclude those used to treat reaction)

D. Reporter (see confidentiality section on first page

16. Name and professional Address:_____

Pin code: _____ E-mail _____

Tel. No. (with STD code): _____

Occupation _____ Signature _____

17. Causality assessment	18. Date of this report (dd/mm/yyyy)

Fig. 4.1

Management of Adverse Drug Reaction

It also seems clear that careful clinical management of a patient, with close monitoring of the patient's responses to manipulation of the drug (s) used, as well as exclusion of more likely causes, can lead to a diagnosis with a high probability of drug causation. This is to be contrasted with epidemiological evidence, which demonstrates a probability based on the incidence in an exposed group versus controls. For rare adverse reactions, the lack of power of some observational studies may be insufficient, and controlled clinical trials may be impracticable because of costs. Individual case information remains very valuable, not in quantitative terms, but in showing high probability that a particular adverse drug effect can indeed happen at least once.

1. **Ensure a complete medical history**
   a. First, it is necessary to be as sure as possible about drug exposure, to avoid diagnostic errors.
   b. If the clinical finding likely to have a subacute or chronic cause, the drug history must go back to a time well before the likely onset of the complaint.
   c. Ask patients about illnesses or symptoms, the patient may have had and find out if they used drugs to manage them. This approach is likely to pick up the use of self-prescribed products, such as over-the-counter drugs and 'alternative' remedies, and the use of other people's drugs.
   d. The patient should be asked specifically about the use of drugs such as oral contraceptives, chronic treatments (always ask about the use of anticoagulants) and also the use of recreational drugs.

2. **Specific tests for adverse drug effects**
   a. There are some diagnostic tests that can be used for adverse reactions/effects. Some may be useful in simply looking for suggestive diagnostic patterns amongst standard tests; for instance, liver function, or perhaps specific histology from biopsied lesions.
   b. For some drugs, there is the possibility of specific drug monitoring to assess whether the drug level in blood, plasma or another body fluid is at a therapeutic, and not toxic level. Such monitoring is available for a variety of drugs with a small difference between therapeutic and toxic levels; a 'low therapeutic index' and is particularly relevant to pharmacologically related adverse reactions.
   c. A more interventional approach is usually needed. Exposure to a suspected drug may be manipulated by altering the dose or discontinuing the drug(s).
   d. Using the timing of the start and discontinuation of treatments in relation to symptoms and signs is a crucial aid to diagnosis.
   e. When several drugs are taken together, and particularly if they are changed at the same time, the diagnosis and management are complicated. Knowing the relative incidence of an adverse drug effect related to the suspect drugs will be helpful.

3. **Drug interaction**
   a. In clinical practice, one often encounters two or more drugs where their pharmacodynamic effects are additive, causing clinical problems.

b. These are often avoidable medication errors. Interactions can also occur with food products that can alter cytochrome P450 (CYP) enzyme function. It is also important to remember disease processes that may alter drug clearance, particularly liver and renal function.

4. Genotyping

a. Genetic tests can determine the susceptibility of individuals and include general tests, such as tests for porphyria and sickle cell anaemia, and specific tests for drug metabolism, such as acetylator status and liver oxidative enzyme status. These tests are also very useful in preventing problems with subsequent drug treatment.

b. There are, however, some examples of the use of genomic data in predicting safe use of drugs, such as the antiretroviral drug abacavir. It has been shown that there is a strong predictive association between this hypersensitivity reaction and HLA-B*5701, indicating that exclusion of HLA-B*5701 positive individuals from abacavir treatment would largely prevent this reaction.

5. Treatment of adverse drug effects

a. When treating an adverse drug reaction, there are two useful guidelines—Do not confuse the clinical picture unnecessarily by using more drugs unless absolutely necessary and have a clear objective for the treatment, carefully monitoring its success or failure, with a general aim of not using the treatment for longer than is necessary.

b. An adverse effect will sometimes produce long-term and even permanent conditions that need treatment. Examples: pulmonary fibrosis, which will usually need corticosteroid and even immunosuppressive therapy, and acute renal and hepatic failure, which may well need supportive therapy and intensive care and even transplant surgery where that is available. Other surgery may sometimes be necessary for sclerotic adverse reactions affecting the skin, lungs or heart.

c. More controversial is the use of two drugs to treat the same condition, both of them in lower than recommended doses for effective treatment, in order to avoid adverse drug effects. It should be emphasized that such an approach should be considered very carefully, and an alternative using a single drug may be preferable.

Some specific antidotes for common drug toxicity

Sr. No.	Drug causing toxicity	Antidote	Dose
1.	Morphine and other opioids	Naloxone	1–2 mg IV repeated every 10–15 minutes
2.	Paracetamol	N-acetyl cysteine	Oral 140 mg/kg followed by 70 mg/kg every 4 hours or IV 150 mg/kg infusion over 15 minutes repeated as required
3.	Heparin	Protamine sulphate	1 mg IV for every 100 units of heparin

Sr. No.	Drug causing toxicity	Antidote	Dose
4.	Cyanide	Sodium nitrate + sodium thiosulfate	10 ml of 3% solution IV, 50 ml of 25% solution IV
5.	Organophosphates	Atropine, oximes	2 mg IV repeated every 10 minutes Pralidoxime 1 gram IV every 3–4 hours 3 doses
6.	Atropine	Physostigmine	1–2 mg IV slowly (or SC) may be repeated if symptoms reappear
7.	Curare and other non-depolarizing skeletal muscle relaxant	Neostigmine	2 mg IV repeated as required
8.	Copper	d-penicillamine	100 mg/kg/day orally in 4 divided doses for 3–7 days
9.	Iron	Desferrioxamine	15 mg/kg/hr IV (100 mg desferri-oxamine binds 8.5 mg of iron
10.	Arsenic	Dimercaprol	1st day 400–800 mg deep IM in divided doses, 2nd and 3rd day 200–400 mg 4th day onwards 100–200 mg
11.	Lead	Calcium disodium edetate day	1 gm in 250 ml saline infusion twice a day
12.	Insulin	Glucose	50 ml of 50% solution
13.	Streptokinase and other fibrinolytics	Epsilon amino caproic acid	5 gm oral IV followed by 1 gm hourly till bleeding stops (max 30 gm in 24 hours)
14.	Digitalis	Digoxin specific antibody fragments	One vial for every 500 mg of digoxin
15.	Nitrates	Methylene blue	0.1% solution slow IV in the dose of 1–2 mg/kg body weight
16.	Carbon monoxide	Oxygen	100% by high-flow non-rebreating mask
17.	Methanol, ethylene glycol	Ethanol or Fomepizole	10% ethanol is given orally 0.7 mg/kg loading dose 0.15 ml/kg infusion, loading dose 15 mg/kg repeated every 12 hours
18.	Warfarin	Vitamin K1 oxide, fresh blood	10 mg IM followed by 5 mg 4 hrly as required
19.	Benzodiazepines	Flumazenil	0.2 mg IV repeated as required (max 3 mg)
20.	Iodine	Sodium thiosulphate	

Pharmacovigilance programme of India

The Central Drugs Standard Control Organization, New Delhi, under the control of Ministry of Health and Family Welfare, Government of India, has initiated a nationwide pharmacovigilance programme. For the Safety of public health in India, the Indian Pharmacopoeia Commission, Ghaziabad (UP), is the national coordinating centre for monitoring adverse drug reaction (ADR). The global ADR monitoring centre

(WHO-Uppsala Monitoring Centre), Sweden, to contribute in the global ADR database. All the NMC approved medical colleges and all government and corporate hospitals will be enrolled in the programme to cover entire nation.

CAUSALITY ASSESSMENT

Causality assessment can be defined as the assessment of relationship between a drug treatment and the occurrence of adverse event. For risk benefit assessment, causality is important, especially when it involves post-marketing safety signals.

The causality assessment system proposed by the World Health Organization Collaborating Center for International Drug Monitoring, the Uppsala Monitoring Center (WHO-UMC) and the Naranjo Probability Scale, are generally accepted and most widely used methods for causal assessment in clinical settings as they deliver a simple methodology. The WHO–UMC causality system quantifies clinical-pharmacological aspects, while previous knowledge of the ADR plays a less prominent role.

Table 4.1: Criteria for causality assessment using WHO-UMC scale

Causality term	Assessment criteria*
Certain	• Event or laboratory test abnormality, with plausible time relationship to drug intake • Cannot be explained by disease or other drugs • Response to withdrawal plausible (pharmacologically/pathologically) • Event definitive pharmacologically or phenomenologically (i.e. an objective and specific medical disorder or a recognised pharmacological phenomenon) • Rechallenge satisfactory, if necessary
Probable/likely	• Event or laboratory test abnormality, with reasonable time relationship to drug intake • Unlikely to be attributed to disease or other drugs • Response to withdrawal clinically reasonable • Rechallenge not required
Possible	• Event or laboratory test abnormality, with reasonable time relationship to drug intake • Could also be explained by disease or other drugs • Information on drug withdrawal may be lacking or unclear
Unlikely	• Event or laboratory test abnormality, with a time to drug intake the makes a relationship improbable (but not impossible) • Disease or other drugs provide plausibe explanations
Conditional/ Unclassified	• Event or laboratory test abnormality • More data for proper assessment needed, or • Additional data under examination
Unassessable/ Unclassifiable	• Report suggesting an adverse reation • Cannot be judged because information is insufficient or contradictory • Data cannot be supplemented or verified

Problem Based Exercise on Adverse Drug Reation

1. **A 30-year-old female reported to a doctor with complaints of weakness and giddiness. On examination, it is found that the patient had pale conjuctiva. Anamia was confirmed with Hb report being 4.5%. The patients was given Inj. Iron Dextran IM. Within few minutes, patients begun complaining of dizziness, palpitation and was sweating profusely.**

   a. What is the likely cause? How could have this adverse effects been prevented?

   Ans: This is a case of hypersentitivity reaction with injection Iron Dextran IM adminstered to correct anemia. Iron-Dextran is antigenic, and anaphylactic reactions are more common with Iron-Dextran than the newer preparations. Taking past history of iron therapy is important. Test dose of Ion-dextran should have been given. A test dose of 0.5 ml Iron-Dextran injected IV over 5–10 min. Injection should be terminated if patient complains of giddiness, paresthesias or tightness in the chest.

2. **A 5-year-old child was brought to a hospital with complaints of diminished hearing. The child had not received any medication previously.**

   What history should be elicited? How can this condition be prevented?

   Ans: Importance of eliciting antenatal history of drug exposure should be emphasized. The mother of child may have received streptomycin in pregnancy giving rise to this problem complaints of diminished hearing. Such condition in children can be prevented if use of teratogenic drugs in pregnant woman is restricted.

3. **An adult female presented with a history of generalised tonic clonic seizure. There was no family history of epilepsy, also no history of any birth injury and no fever. On examination, there was no neurological abnormality. EEG was suggestive of primary generalised seizures. The lady was started on phenytoin therapy 100 mg TDS and was asked to follow up 2 weeks later and keep record of the number of seizures.**

   a. She comes back with complaints of 4 seizures in the past fortnight. How will you proceed?

   Ans: Since the woman complains of 4 seizures in the past fortnight history of patient complaints should be elicited and the therapeutic drug level of Phenytoin should be measured.

   b. 2 weeks later she now comes with giddiness and unsteady gait. Her plasma phenytoin level is 24 µg/ml. What will you do now?

Ans: Giddiness with unsteady gait are the adverse aspects of phenytoin since the plasma phenytoin levels of 24 µg/ml, is more than therapeutic index level. So the reduction in dose is required.

> **c. The lady comes back 6 months later with history of amenorrhoea for 2 month. Preganancy is detected. What will be your decision?**

Ans: Most of anti-epileptic drugs are teratogenic. However anti-epileptic drug therapy in pregnancy should not be stopped because there is a high risk of developing convulsions on stoppage of drugs during pregnancy. These can cause birth defects and mental retardation in offspring. It should be told to the patient that phenytoin induced teratogenesis is very low and benefit of continuing anti-epileptic drug outways the risk. Carbamazipine is avoided as it is expensive. Phenytoin and phenobarbitol are prescribed more commonly.

4. **A young women was prescribed Tab. Nimesulide 1 tablets once daily for one week for backache. 5 days later she developed weakness and arthralgia. Following this she developed nausea and had two episodes of haematemesis. Later on there was clouding of consciousness, she was brought to the hospital where investigation revealed severe hepatocellular damage. The patient died 2 days later. How will you report this reaction?**

Ans: In this patient, hepatitis has occurred due to Nimesulide. This is rare ADR often there in paucity of data available with the new drug. ADR are detected during post-marketing. The doctor is expected to report the ADR to ADR monitoring centre. The details of patient, the reaction, therapy administered, any other drug taken by patient in the course of A/E and treatment given for same. Details of whether the reaction continued or stopped on cessation of drug therapy and its casual relation to drug needs to be reported. All this data should be submitted by doctor with his registration number.

5. **A 10 year old suffering from pulmonary tuberculosis was prescribed isoniazid + rifampicin + pyrazinamide + ethambutol for 2 months. After 1 month, the child complained of diminished vision.**

> **a. What was the possible cause?**

Ans: This is case of optic neuritis with ethambutol.

> **b. What precaution to be taken while prescribing in a paediatric population?**

Ans: Ethambutol should not be ideally prescribed in prediatric population.

6. **This child was prescribed an oral medication for the management of a congenital disorder. Three months later, the child came with puffiness of face. A diagnosis of "moon face" was made.**

> **a. Mention the name of the drug that has caused the adverse drug reaction?**

Ans: Presenting disorder, i.e. congenital autoimmune disease

ADR: Moon face

Probable drug: Corticosteroid such as Prednisolone and Dexamethasone.

7. **A 55-years-old execuitve with congestive cardiac failure on therapy came back two months later with complaints of gynaecomastia.**

a. **Which of the drug is likely to cause this adverse effects in this patient?**

Ans: Digitalis

8. **A 40-years-old man came with swollen lips after taking an antihypertensive for the treatment of hypertension. A diagnosis of angioedema was made.**

    a. **Name the antihypertensive agent?**

Ans: ACE inhibitor—Captropil

    b. **Which can cause the above side effects?**

Ans: Swollen lips caused because of angioedema mainly by ACE inhibitor: Enalapril.

    c. **Name other drug, which can cause this side effects?**

Ans: Cephalosporin

9. **A patient is prescribed insulin-therapy. After 3 years he reports to your OPD with complaints that he has developed "pits" in his thighs.**

    a. **What is diagnosis?**

Ans: Insulin induced lipodystropy.

    b. **What important instruction should have been given to avoid this condition?**

Ans: Take all medicines regularly, rotate the site of insulin injection.

10. **A 25-year-old woman came to the OPD with complaints of a lesion on the skin. On inquiry mentioned that she was taking treatment for an upper respiratory tract infection for the past 3 days, diagnosis of fixed drug eruption is made.**

    a. **Mention the drugs likely to cause this ADR ?**

Ans: Drugs: Sulphonamides, Phenytoin, Quinidine, ACE inhibitor

ADR: Lesion on skin fixed the eruption.

11. **A 40-year-old female came to the OPD with complaints of excessive hair growth on the face. On inquiry she mentioned that she was taking antihypertensive medication for the treatment of her high blood pressure for past one year.**

    a. **Mention the drug likely to cause the above side effects?**

Ans: Antihypertensive drug associated with ADR: excessive hair growth on face: Minoxidil. Other drugs causing excessive hair growth: Glucocorticoids, Cyclosporin

12. **A patient suffering from tonsilar diptheria (culture +ve) was treated with erythromycin. Three weeks after treatment, patient has developed fever, lymphadenopathy, eosinophilia.**

    a. **What is the name of this ADR?**

Ans: ADR: Fixed drug eruption

Probable drug: Penicilin, Cephalosprin.

13. **A child with vomiting was given an injection to stop vomiting. He developed abnormal movements of face and neck.**

    a. **What is the cause for the new manifestations?**

Ans: To control vomiting, the child was given an injection of metoclopramide, knows as an antiemetic drug, known to cause extrapyramidal symptoms that generally manifest as acute dystonic reactions within the initial 24–48 hours of use. Metoclopramide can cause these se2vere adverse events; acute dystonic reaction, and therefore should be used with caution in children. The drug should be immediately withdrawn.

14. **Patient of bronchial asthma receiving some inhalational medication develops oral candidiasis. Identify likely agent and how this could have been prevented?**

Ans: Inhaled steroids such as Fluticasone Propionate and Beclomethasone Dipropionate play a central role in the treatment of bronchial asthma. They are known to cause oral candidiasis as an adverse effect. Gargling with dilution of Antifungals (amphotericin B/Nystatin) is effective in treating oral candidiasis among asthmatic patients treated with inhaled steroids.

15. **A pediatric patient, aged 5 years old, suffering from productive cough. He was given cough expectorant containing Salbutamol 2 mg and Guaiphenesin 100 mg/10 ml. Child develops severe tremors in hand.**

    a. Which is the drug responsible for development of tremors in hand?
Ans: Salbutamol is the responsible drug for development of tremors in hand.

    b. What could be probable mechanism for the induction of tremors?
Ans: Salbutamol by its action on pre synaptic Beta 2 receptors increases the release of acetylcholine from cholinergic somatic nerve causing tremors.

    c. How will you overcome salbutamol-induced tremors?
Ans: Withdrawal of salbutamol containing expectorant is essential.

16. **An executive suffering from moderate hypertension was prescribed nifedipine, enalapril and hydrochlorothiazide for the management of hypertension. He develops a persistent brassy cough after a week.**

    a. Which is the antihypertensive agent causing cough?
Ans: ACE inhibitor enalapril is known to produce a persistent cough within 1–8 weeks of therapy.

    b. What could be probable mechanism for development of cough?
Ans: Development of cough is caused by inhibition of breakdown of bradykinin/substance P in the lungs of susceptible individuals.

    c. Which is the alternative drug available for management of hypertension in this patient?
Ans: Angiotensin 2 receptor blockers such as losartan, candesertan, irbesertan can be given in this patient as alternative antihypertensive agents

17. **A male patient working in office used to get sneezing every day morning. He has been prescribed promethazine and advised not to drive a vehicle or operate heavy machinery.**

    a. What is the side effect of promethazine?
Ans: Promethazine causes sedation.

b. What could be the reason for the development of such side effect?

Ans: Histaminergic H1 receptors in the CNS are blocked by Promethazine and sedation is induced.

c. Which is the alternative antihistaminic available for sneezing?

Ans: Alternative non-sedative antihistaminic Cetirizine or Levo Cetirizine can be given to patient having sneezing

18. **A male patient was suffering from malaria and was treated with chloroquine. He develops severe nausea and vomiting for which he has been given injection metoclopramide, but he developed tremors and rigidity.**

    a. What is the cause of development of tremors and rigidity?

    Ans: Metoclopramide causes extra pyramidal effects-parkinsonism like symptoms, e.g. tremors and rigidity, due to Dopaminergic D2—receptor blockade in basal ganglia.

    b. How will you manage tremors and rigidity induced by metoclopramide?

    Ans: 1. Withdraw Metoclopramide
    2. Give centrally acting anticholinegic Trihexyphenidyl HCL to overcome the side effects caused by Metoclopramide.

19. **An elderly male patient aged 55-years-old was suffering from benign prostatic hyperplasia (BPH) and treated with Prazosin Hydrochloride 1 mg twice day. He develops dizziness and fainting.**

    a. With could be the cause of dizziness and fainting?

    Ans: Prazosin produces Orthostatic hypotension producing dizziness and fainting.

    b. What could be the mechanism for the adverse effect of prazosin?

    Ans: Prazosin blocks selectively postsynaptic α_{-1} receptors of vascular smooth muscles of both resistance and capacitance vessels. Therefore, prazosin produces vasodilatation, resulting into orthostatic hypotension.

    c. Which is the alternative drug available in replacement of prazosin for benign prostatic hyperplasia (BPH)?

    Ans: Tamsulosin uroselective α_{1A} blocker available for BPH. It blocks selectively α_{1A} subtype in the bladder base and prostate without affecting α_{1B} of vascular smooth muscle. Therefore does not produce orthostatic hypotension.

20. **A 50-years-old male patient suffering from angina has been prescribed Tab. Isosorbide dinitrate. After a weak, patient felt dizziness and weakness. For which he withdraws the therapy.**

    a. What are the adverse effects responsible for the withdrawal of therapy by the patient.

    Ans: Patients desires to withdraw antianginal therapy due to certain isosorbide dinitrate–induced adverse effects like throbbing headache, hypotension and reflex tachycardia.

    b. What could be the mechanism of action for the development of such adverse effects of isosorbide dinitrate.

Ans: Isosorbide dinitrate produces sudden fall in blood pressure due to vasodilation and reflex tachycardia. Throbbing headache is also due to vasodilatation at meningeal blood vessels.

c. What could be the alternative therapeutic approach for the management of angina.

Ans: Cardioselective receptor blocker–Metoprolol should be given along with isosorbide dinitrate to patients as prophylactive therapy so that dose of isosorbide dinitrate can be reduced.

Identify and Describe the Management of Drug Interactions

INTRODUCTION

A drug interaction occurs when a patient's response to a drug is modified by food, nutritional supplements, formulated excipients, environmental factors, other drugs or disease. Interactions between drugs (drug-drug interactions) may be beneficial or harmful. Harmful drug-drug interactions are important as they cause 10–20% of the adverse drug reactions requiring hospitalization and they can be avoided. Thus, identification and management of drug-drug interaction and how to manage them is an important part of clinical practice.

Types of Drug-Drug Interactions

a. Pharmaceutic drug—Drug interactions occur when the formulation of one drug is altered by another before it is administered. For example, precipitation of sodium thiopentone and vecuronium within an intravenous giving set.

b. Pharmacokinetic drug—Drug interactions occur when one drug changes the systemic concentration of another drug, altering 'how much' and for 'how long' it is present at the site of action.

c. Pharmacodynamic drug—Drug interactions occur when interacting drugs have either additive effects in which case the overall effect is increased, or opposing effects in which case the overall effect is decreased or even 'cancelled out'.

How to Identify Drug-Drug Interactions in Clinical Practice

1. Eliciting a full drug history including over-the-counter and herbal products.
2. Prescribe few drugs and know them well.
3. Drugs with a narrow therapeutic index are particularly susceptible to pharmacokinetic drug-drug interactions (Table 6.1).
4. A small number of drugs are important 'perpetrators' of pharmacokinetic drug-drug interactions.
5. Monitoring patients for drug toxicity or loss of efficacy is part of routine care. Checking for changes in symptoms, biomarkers of effect, or drug concentrations soon after prescription changes.
6. Knowledge of resources for drug-drug interaction.
   a. Individual drug monographs in formularies
   b. Online reference database, e.g. Stockley's drug Interactions and Micromedex
7. Prescribing and dispensing software.

Management of Drug-Drug Interaction

1. Patient education via verbal instruction from healthcare provider, patient instruction leaflets.
2. Adoption of therapeutic drug monitoring protocols in susceptible patients (e.g. elderly people with multiple comorbidities) and drugs with narrow therapeutic index.
3. Discontinuation if possible the drug causing the interaction, or the drug affected by the interaction. Alternatives might be to decrease the dose, or change time of administration.
4. Substitution of the suspected drug with another drug of similar efficacy but lower potential for interactions.
5. Review all drugs in the active profile for appropriate indications and target a lowest effective dose.

Table 6.1: Examples of drug classes containing several narrow therapeutic index drugs

Drug class	Example
Antiarrhythmics	Amiodarone
Anticoagulants	Warfarin
Antiepileptics	Phenytoin
Antineoplastics	Sunitinib
Aminoglycoside antibiotics	Gentamicin
Immunosuppressants	Tacrolimus

SOME IMPORTANT DRUG–DRUG INTERACTION

1. Fluoxetine and Phenelzine

The interaction can result in a central serotonin syndrome. This condition is characterized by mental status change, agitation, diaphoresis, tachycardia, and death. These symptoms can develop quickly with only 1 or 2 doses of fluoxetine when combined with phenelzine. Serotonin syndrome is possible with any monoamine oxidase inhibitor (MAOI), such as phenelzine or tranylcypromine sulfate, in combination with any drug that increases serotonin levels, such as dextromethorphan, meperidine, and other selective serotonin reuptake inhibitors.

2. Digoxin and Quinidine

The interaction can lead to a marked increase in plasma concentration levels of digoxin in more than 90% of patients. Significant changes in serum digoxin are noticed within 24 hours. The average increase is roughly 2-fold. The effects from this interaction range from nausea and vomiting to death. The primary mechanism for this interaction is a decreased volume of distribution of digoxin, secondary to its displacement from binding sites in body tissues. Quinidine also decreases renal and nonrenal excretion rates of digoxin, which leads to increased steady-state concentrations of the cardiac glycoside. Ideally, patients taking digoxin should avoid the use of quinidine.

3. Sildenafil and Isosorbide Mononitrate

Sildenafil may markedly increase the hypotensive effects of isosorbide mononitrate. More than 100 deaths have been reported since 1998, when sildenafil was made available in the United States. Most deaths were among patients with 1 or more risk factors, including obesity, hypertension, and cigarette smoking. Sildenafil was developed as a phosphodiesterase-5 (PDE5) inhibitor. In the presence of PDE5 inhibitors, nitrates can cause intense increases in cyclic guanosine monophosphate and dramatic drops in blood pressure. Patients taking isosorbide mononitrate or any nitrate, including nitroglycerin, should be advised not to take sildenafil.

4. Potassium Chloride and Spironolactone

The combination may result in hyperkalemia. The resulting hyperkalemia can be serious and may lead to cardiac failure and death. Patients with renal impairment are especially prone to this effect. Spironolactone is a competitive antagonist of mineral corticoids, of which aldosterone is a potent example. This mechanism occurs in the kidney at the distal portion of the nephron and leads to the excretion of sodium ions while saving potassium ions. Patients receiving potassium-depleting diuretics, such as amiloride or triamterene, may also experience this interaction. These diuretics can interact with all absorbable forms of potassium bicarbonate, citrate, acetate, gluconite, and iodide salts. Severe hyperkalemia is dangerous, and thus patients who are prescribed spironolactone must undergo an evaluation of serum potassium levels.

5. Clonidine and Propranolol

A sudden withdrawal of clonidine from adjunctive therapy with propranolol may cause fatal rebound hypertension. Clonidine is a central alpha-2 adrenergic agonist that suppresses the sympathetic nervous system from the brain. This activity leads to a decrease in the norepinephrine amounts available in the synaptic cleft of the adrenergic neuron. Alpha-1 receptors then become sensitized because of less norepinephrine available in the cleft. When clonidine is suddenly withdrawn, the result is a large increase in norepinephrine in the synaptic cleft of the adrenergic neuron. The sensitized alpha-1 receptors are stimulated, leading to an exaggerated vasoconstriction. The body cannot compensate for this response because the beta-2 receptors are blocked when a patient is concurrently taking propranolol. Within 24 to 72 hours, a dramatic rebound hypertension is noticed.

6. Warfarin and Diclofenac

Nonsteroidal anti-inflammatory drugs (NSAIDs), such as diflunisal, have been shown to increase the risk for gastrointestinal bleeding and the anticoagulant response of warfarin. Other NSAIDs such as ketoprofen, piroxicam, sulindac, diclofenac, and ketorolac have been shown to have similar interactions with warfarin. Because the interaction between warfarin and diflunisal can lead to GI bleeding or even fatal hemorrhaging, an alternative to diflunisal is suggested. Acetaminophen is the alternative of choice.

7. Theophylline and Ciprofloxacin

The hepatic metabolism of theophylline is inhibited by ciprofloxacin via cytochrome P-450 enzyme system. Theophylline is metabolized by CYP1A2 and to a lesser extent by CYP3A4. Ciprofloxacin and other drugs, including clarithromycin, erythromycin, fluvoxamine, and cimetidine, are all potent inhibitors of CYP1A2. Because they have little effect on CYP1A2, levofloxacin or ofloxacin should be considered as an alternative to ciprofloxacin.Theophylline toxicity is a serious condition; several deaths have been linked with serum concentrations as low as 25 µg/ml.

8. Methotrexate and Probenecid

When probenecid is administered with antineoplastic doses of methotrexate, the result can be a 2- to 3-fold increase in methotrexate levels. Probenecid acts as an active tubular secretion inhibitor and prevents methotrexate from being excreted, thus potentially causing toxicity. This interaction with methotrexate also occurs with penicillins (e.g. amoxicillin, carbenicillin) and salicylates. The risk with low-dose methotrexate (commonly used for arthritis) is lower; in fact, NSAIDs in combination with low-dose methotrexate are often prescribed purposely. Possible alternatives include acetaminophen, as opposed to salicylates or NSAIDs. Celecoxib does not affect methotrexate pharmacokinetics and could be an alternative.

DANGEROUS FOOD DRUG INTERACTION

Does it matter if I take a medicine on a full or empty stomach?

Yes, with some medicines. Some medicines can work faster, slower, better, or worse when you take them on a full or empty stomach. On the other hand, some medicines will upset your stomach, and if there is food in your stomach, that can help reduce the upset. If you don't see directions on your medicine labels, ask your doctor or pharmacist if it is best to take your medicines on an empty stomach (one hour before eating, or two hours after eating), with food, or after a meal (full stomach).

Does it matter if I take my medicine with alcohol?

Yes, the way your medicine works can change when:

    a. You swallow your medicine with alcohol.
    b. You drink alcohol after you've taken your medicine.
    c. You take your medicine after you've had alcohol to drink.
    Alcohol can also add to the side effects caused by medicines.

IMPORTANT FOOD DRUG INTERACTION

1. Warfarin and Vitamin K

Warfarin (Coumadin) is a blood-thinning medication that helps treat and prevent blood clots. Eating certain foods, especially those rich in vitamin K, can diminish warfarin's effectiveness. The highest concentrations of vitamin K are found in green leafy vegetables such as kale, collards, spinach, turnip greens, Brussels sprouts, broccoli, scallions, asparagus, and endive.

2. Insulin, Oral Diabetic Agents, and Alcohol

An alcoholic drink can increase or prolong the effects of insulin or oral diabetic agents and thus lead to hypoglycemia or low blood sugar. The glucose-lowering action of alcohol can last as long as eight to 12 hours. Symptoms of hypoglycemia include nervousness, sweating, trembling, intense hunger, weakness, palpitations, confusion, drowsiness, and ultimately coma. Certain oral diabetic medications such as chlorpropamide can cause dizziness, flushing, and nausea when taken along with alcohol.

3. Digoxin, High-Fiber Diets, and Herbs

Digoxin is used to strengthen the contraction of the heart muscle, slow the heart rate, and promote the elimination of fluid from body tissues. Dietary fiber, specifically insoluble fiber such as wheat bran, can slow down the absorption of digoxin and lessen its effectiveness. To prevent this, elders should take digoxin at least one hour before or two hours after eating a meal. Herb use can also affect digoxin. For example, ginseng can elevate blood levels of digoxin by as much as 75%, while St. John's Wort decreases blood levels of this drug by 25%.

4. Statins and Grapefruit

Statins are highly effective cholesterol-lowering drugs. Drinking grapefruit juice or eating fresh grapefruit can increase the amount of some statins in your blood and lead to potentially greater side effects of these drugs. Side effects of statins include muscle soreness and liver abnormalities reflected in high transaminase levels (serum glutamic-oxaloacetic transaminase and serum glutamic pyruvic transaminase) on a blood test.

5. Calcium Channel Blockers and Grapefruit

Calcium channel blockers are prescribed for high blood pressure. A natural element found in grapefruit latches onto the intestinal enzyme called CYP3A4, which alters the breakdown of the calcium channel blockers, possibly resulting in excessively high blood levels of the drug, along with an increased risk of serious side effects. It doesn't take a jumbo serving of grapefruit to produce a deleterious effect either. For example, a single 6-ounce glass of juice can reduce levels of CYP3A4 by nearly 50%. This effect dissipates slowly. One study indicated that one third of the impact on CYP3A4 from grapefruit juice was still evident a full 24 hours later. The interaction between grapefruit and calcium channel blockers is strongest, for example, with felodipine, nicardipine and amlodipine,diltiazem and nifedipine.

6. Erectile Dysfunction Drugs and Grapefruit

Although unproven, evidence points to the likely fact that grapefruit juice gives a boost to blood levels of erectile dysfunction drugs such as sildenafil (Viagra). This may seem like a boon to some men, but it could trigger headache symptomatic of fatal or near fatal conditions, flushing, or low blood pressure.

7. Acetaminophen and Alcohol

The over-the-counter pain reliever acetaminophen and alcohol don't mix. Two or more alcoholic drinks per day can increase the liver toxicity. This toxicity can happen even if a patient takes less than the maximum 4 grams, or eight tablets. This interaction can be especially problematic in older adults, since the liver's ability to diminish drugs decreases with age.

8. Antibiotics and Dairy Products

Dairy products such as milk, yogurt, and cheese can delay or prevent the absorption of antibiotics such as tetracyclines and ciprofloxacin. This occurs because the calcium in such foods binds to the antibiotics in the stomach and upper small intestine to form an insoluble compound. To avoid problems, it recommends taking an antibiotic one hour before or two hours after a meal. However, there's no need to avoid milk and dairy with all antibiotics.

9. MAOIs and Tyramine-Containing Foods

Monoamine oxidase inhibitors are an older type of antidepressant still prescribed, foods containing tyramines, such as some red wines, malt beer, smoked fish, aged cheeses, and dried fruits, can cause a hypertensive crisis or severe and dangerous elevation in blood pressure when taken with this class of antidepressants.

10. Antithyroid Drugs and Iodine-Rich Foods

Antithyroid drugs are compounds that interfere with the body's production of thyroid hormones, thereby reducing the symptoms of hyperthyroidism. Antithyroid drugs work by preventing iodine absorption in the stomach. A high-iodine diet requires higher doses of antithyroid drugs. The higher the dose of antithyroid drugs, the greater the incidence of side effects that include rashes, hives, and liver disease.

11. Bisphosphonates (Bone Calcium-Phosphorus Metabolism) with Food

Bisphosphonates prevent and treat osteoporosis, a condition in which the bones become thin and weak and break easily. Example, alendronate sodium and alendronate sodium + cholecalciferol are medicines work only when you take them on an empty stomach. Take the medicine (first thing) in the morning with a full glass (six to eight ounces) of plain water while you are sitting or standing up. Don't take with mineral water. Don't take antacids or any other medicine, food, drink, calcium, or any vitamins or other dietary supplements for at least 30 minutes after taking alendronate. Don't lie down for at least 30 minutes after taking alendronate. Don't lie down until you eat your first food of the day.

12. Bronchodilator with Food and Alcohol

Food can have different effects on different forms of theophylline (some forms are regular release, sustained release, and sprinkles). Check with your pharmacist to be sure you know which form of the medicine you use. Follow directions for sprinkle forms of the medicine. You can swallow sprinkle capsules whole or open them and sprinkle them on soft foods, such as applesauce or pudding. Swallow the mixture without chewing, as soon as it is mixed. Follow with a full glass of cool water or juice.

Avoid alcohol if you're using theophylline medicines because alcohol can increase the chance of side effects, such as nausea, vomiting, headache, and irritability.

Problem Based Exercise on Drug Interaction

Exercise 1: Mr. XYZ, aged 60 years, developed idiopathic parkinsonism for which he was prescribed tablets levodopa, 250 mg three times a day after food. During the 6 months of treatment he reported improvement in general condition, reduction in muscle rigidity and tremors.

However, for the past 15 days, he has noticed rigidity and tremors, though he was taking levodopa. On taking a detailed history, he revealed that he was taking multivitamin tablets, which some doctor had given him as a free sample.

a. What could be drug interaction?

Ans. Pyridoxine (vitamin B6) available in multivitamin tablets increases decarboxylation of levodopa in the periphery, resulting into a decrease concentration of levodopa in the central nervous system.

The drug interaction between Levodopa and pyridoxine causes the appearance of rigidity and tremors showing failure of therapy even with Levodopa.

b. How will you overcome this drug interaction?

Ans. Withdrawal of multivitamin tablets containing pyridoxine is necessary. Dopa decarboxylase inhibitor carbidopa should be given along with levodopa for the improvement of clinical response.

Exercise 2: Mrs. ABC, a known hypertensive for the past 5 years was on hydrochlorothiazide along with other antihypertensive drug. She was started on digoxin 0.25 mg/day for the treatment of mild CCF.

a. What drug interaction would you suspect if she develops ectopic beats and tachyarrhythmia?

Ans: The drug interaction between diuretic hydrochlorothiazide and digoxin causes cardiac arrhythmias, i.e. Ectopic beats and Tachyarrhythmia.

b. What could be the mechanism for this drug interaction?

Ans: Hydrochlorothiazide causes hypokalemia. A decrease in K^+ level in plasma produces more binding of digoxin leads to digoxin toxicity. Inhibition of Na^+–K^+ ATPase (Na^+ pump) by digitalis causes accumulation of intracellular Na^+ and Ca^{++} resulting into arrhythmias.

Exercise 3: Mr. ABC, who was a chronic alcoholic, voluntarily opted for de-addiction. He was hospitalized and was put on disulfiram 500 mg a day. Ten days later, when he was allowed to go home for a brief visit in the evening, he could not control himself and consumed alcohol.

a. What signs and symptoms do you expect in this patient?

Ans: Chronic alcoholic patient on disulfiram therapy with consumption of alcohol develops: nausea, vomiting, flushing, hypotension, palpitation, perspiration, headache, mental confusion and circulatory collapse.

b. What is the underlying mechanism?

Ans: Disulfiram irreversibly inhibits aldehyde dehydrogenase and causes accumulation of aldehyde which is responsible for development of above-mentioned signs and symptoms.

c. Can this interaction develops with drugs other than disulfiram? If yes, name such drugs.

Ans: Yes. This reaction can develop with drugs other than disulfiram like: Metronidazole, Sulfonylureas, Cephalosporins.

Exercise 4: An adult patient aged 40 years suffering from COPD due to bronchitis has been treated with following therapy.

℞

Tab. Salbutamol	4 mg	TDS
Cap. Theophylline SR	400 mg	BD
Tab. Ciprofloxacin	500 mg	BD

Patient develops severe toxicities like: Dyspepsia, gastric pain, headache, delirium worsening cardiovascular status due to drug interaction.

a. What could be the drug interaction in the present therapeutic approach?

Ans: Ciprofloxacin inhibits the metabolism of theophylline and increases its plasma level. Therefore, these two drugs given concurrently developed drug interaction.

b. Which is the drug to be avoided?

Ans: Ciprofloxacin can be avoided to treat bronchitis in this case. Amoxycillin or cefadroxil can be given in patients having COPD associated with bronchitis.

c. How will you manage this drug interaction?

Ans : Alternatively, the dose of theophylline should be reduced to 2/3.

Critical Appraisal of Drug Promotional Literature

INTRODUCTION

According to the World Health Organisation (WHO) medicinal drug promotion is defined as "all informational and persuasive activities by manufacturers and distributors, the effect of which is to induce the prescription, supply, purchase, and/or use of medicinal drugs." Therefore, for the rational use of drugs, WHO has laid down ethical criteria for medicinal drug promotion and has recommended pharmaceutical industries to implement these guidelines.

The drug advertisements should contain the following information:

1. Name of each active ingredient, as either the international nonproprietary name (INN) or the approved generic name, in addition to the brand name of the product.
2. Legal category (e.g. prescription or nonprescription, narcotic or other controlled status).
3. Composition, that is, content of active ingredient per dose or concentration.
4. Name of other ingredients (excipients) known to cause problems.
5. Approved indications.
6. Dosing regimens for these indications, with reference to special situations (e.g. children, pregnancy, lactation, renal impairment, etc.) as appropriate.
7. Adverse drug reactions and interactions, with an indication of their frequency.
8. Special precautions and contraindications in use.
9. Reference to scientific literature, as appropriate.
10. Name and address of the manufacturer or distributor.

Note that the manufacturers are free and expected to incorporate any additional relevant information, such as pharmacokinetic information, special storage or handling requirements, overdose management and commercial packaging information.

Drug advertisements are used as a tool for drug promotion because the pharmaceutical manufacturers wish their drugs to be prescribed as widely as possible. Advertisements are necessary as they provide information to the doctors about the newly released preparations in the market, new uses for existing medicines and properties of medicines. But unfortunately, because pharmaceutical sales is a full fledged commercial activity, the pharmaceutical industry is not driven by altruistic motives. Profit is the major driving force for such activities. This profit motive makes pharmaceutical companies prone to unethical promotional practices at times and induce them to take advantage of regulatory lapses to enhance their sales mostly through excessive and irrational use of medicines.

To achieve this goal, the product leaflets, brochures, flyers are prepared in such a way that they look attractive and are continuously bombarded on the physician's mind. As a result of this, the prescribers who don't pay conscious attention to the facts are liable to be influenced by the way the advertisers intend, leading to a change in their prescribing behaviour. On the other hand, those who examine it critically will learn what they want. However, a majority of the prescribers in India lack knowledge on the critical evaluation of drug promotional literature because they are not trained on this aspect during the medical curriculum or later. That is why the critical appraisal of drug literature is very important for undergraduate practicals.

Critically appraising promotional literature provided by pharmaceutical companies:

1. The generic name must appear prominently in comparison to the proprietary or brand name. Brand name is larger than the generic name with unique lettering and colouring style but there is no mention of the corresponding generic anywhere.
2. Efficacy and safety claims should be on the basis of measurable clinical outcomes which are of greatest relevance to the physicians. Very often surrogate end points are used which do not correlate well with meaningful clinical outcome.
3. Claims should be balancing both benefits and risks. Marketing claims highlight beneficial effects of their products with too little emphasis on potential harm.
4. The cost aspect of the drug is frequently highlighted in drug advertisements. Misleading information about economic benefits can easily lead to doctors over prescribing more expensive medicines that do not offer any additional clinical benefit.
5. Unscientific tables and graphs.
6. Wordings and illustrations should be fully consistent with approved scientific data sheet for the drug. The word 'safe' to be used if properly qualified. Even with peer reviewed papers, only those that support rather than contradict claims, may be selectively cited.
7. Images often used in promotional literature to supplement frankly misleading claims

Drug Promotional Literature Checksheet

1. Deviations/deficiencies vis-a-vis sample drug information sheet.
2. Objectionable figures.
3. Unscientific tables and graphs.
4. Irrelevant references.
5. Compare letter size of generic name and brand name.

Objectives for Students

Analyse critically drug promotional literature for proprietary preparations in terms of the following:

1. Pharmacological actions of their ingredients.
2. Claims of pharmaceutical companies.
3. Economics of use.
4. Rational or irrational nature of fixed dose drug combinations.
5. Identify and get sensitized to unethical marketing practices by pharmaceuticals.
6. Realize the extent to which drug advertisements can influence prescribing behavior.

New Drug Discovery

Drug development is considered as a series of well defined steps, culminating if successful in market authorization of the drug. Drug discovery is the process of identifying compound that have the potential to become useful new therapies.

Earlier majority of drug developed or discovered by random screening or serendipity. Now-a-days, mostly the drug are synthesized by recombinant DNA technology or modifying the structure of existing drug. The drug discovery process comprises following research activity.

1. **Serendipitous discovery of drug:**
    a. Discovery by chance is called serendipitous discovery.
    b. Several examples are there that drug is developed for some purpose in a planned way and it has been found that this drug has other effects.
    c. Discovery of penicillin was a by-chance discovery.
    d. Phenytoin was synthesized as sedative-hypnotic but it lacks sedation and after many years, it was found that phenytoin has anticonvulsant effects.
2. **Target identification:** Drugs usually act on the cellular or genetic composition of the body called as targets and it is associated with disease and molecules has identified which have interaction with targets which will helpful to treat disease.
3. **Target validation:** It is the process by which predicted molecular target. For example, protein or nucleic acid of a small molecule verified. Target validation can include, determination of the structure activity relationship of analogs of the small molecule, generating a drug resistant mutant of the presumed target.
4. **Lead identification:** The result of target validation stage can assist in lead compound identification. Lead compounds are chemical compounds that show desired biological or pharmacological activity and may iniate the development of new clinically relevant compounds. These are typically used as starting points in drug design to give new drug entities.
5. **Lead optimization:** It compares the properties of various lead compounds and provides information to help pharmaceutical and biotechnological companies.
6. **High throughput screening:** It is an automated system that test small amounts of large number of compounds against potential targets. Development of quality leads compounds using hit confirmation and to lead approach.

7. **Combinatorial chemistry:** This comprises chemical–synthetic methods that make it possible to prepare a large number (tens to thousands or even millions) of compounds in a single process. These compound libraries can be made as mixtures, sets of individual compounds or chemical structures generated by

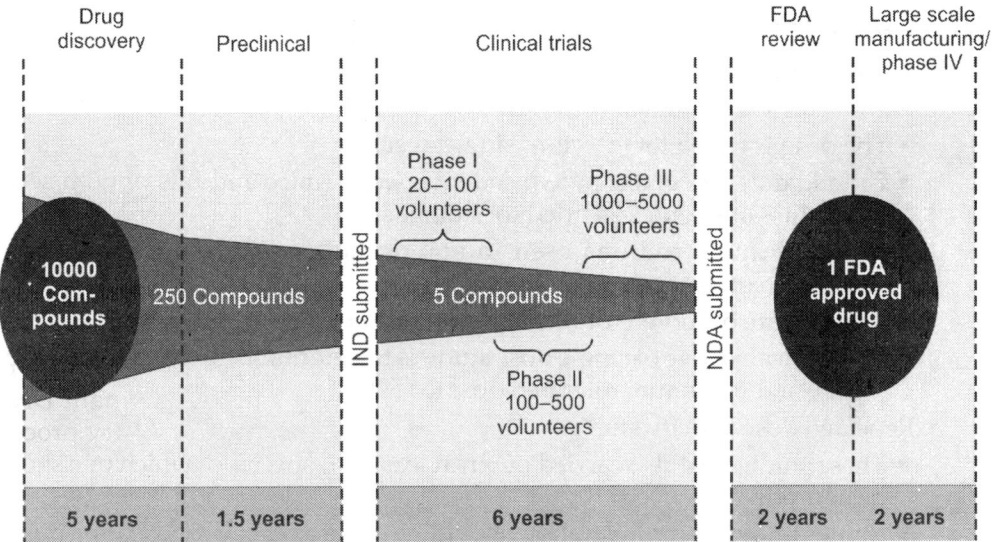

Fig. 9.1: **Schematic showing** various phases during drug discovery

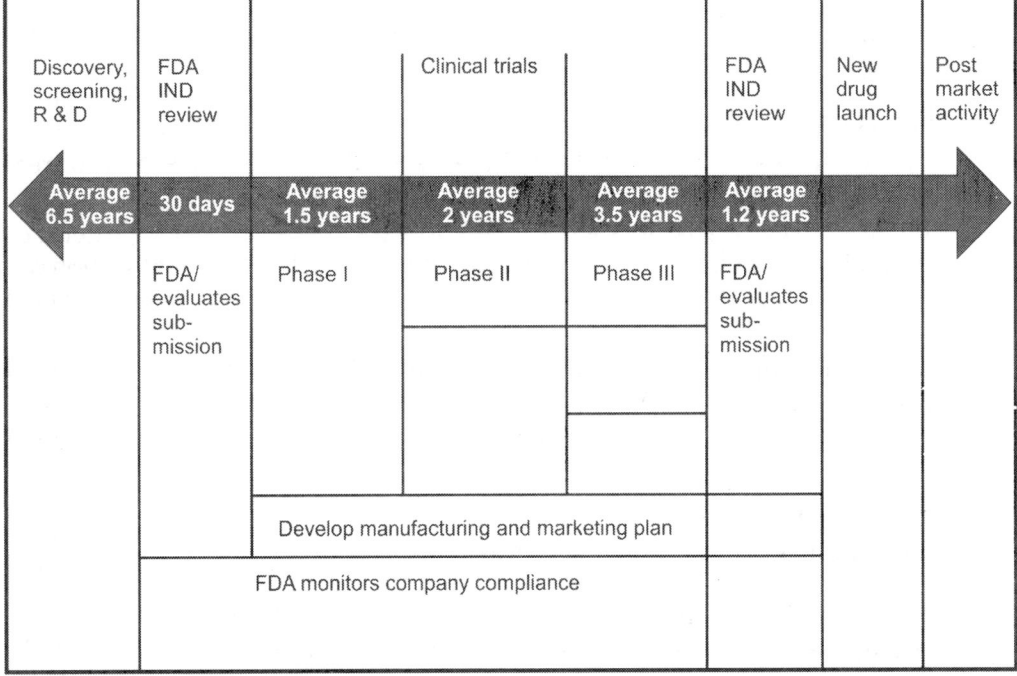

Fig. 9.2: **Schematic showing** process of a new drug development

computer software. Combinatorial chemistry can be used for the synthesis of small molecules and for peptides.

8. **Biochemistry/microbiology assay:** Several enzyme based assay, receptor radio ligand binding assay are used in drug discovery process.

Preclinical Studies

1. **Systemic toxicity studies**

   a. Acute/single dose toxicity studies
   - The drug is tested for effects of single dose.
   - Graded dose are given in two rodent species (mice and rats of both sexes) using the same route intended for humans.
   - One additional route is used in one of the species to ensure systemic absorption of the drug.
   - Animals are observed for mortality for upto 14 days.
   - The main objective of single dose study is to determine minimum lethal dose (MLD) and maximum tolerated dose (MTD).

   b. Repeated dose toxicity studies
   - These studies are also carried out in at least two species of which one should be nonrodent.
   - Routes of drug administration should be same as that proposed for human use.
   - Three doses are selected for study.
     - Highest dose having observable toxicity.
     - Mid dose causing some symptoms but no gross toxicity or death.
     - Lowest dose free of toxicity and comparable to the intended therapeutic dose.

2. **Subacute and chronic toxicity studies**
   - The drug administered for longer period ranging from 1 week to 2 years, sometime for life time of the animals.
   - Small animals such as mice and rats are used for this purpose.
   - To find out, the effects of drug which are not manifested after single dose.
   - To mimic the condition in which the drug is likely to be used in human being as far as possible.
   - To ascertain the safety of drug in the form of sufficient evidences.

3. **Test for local irritation effect:** The drug should be tested in the dosage form in which it is intended to be used in human beings such as oral, parenteral, topical including ocular, vaginal and rectal.

4. **Special toxicological effects**

   a. **Effect on reproduction:** The studies are conducted on rats and drug is administered before and after the mating period to investigate mating behavior, fertility, effects of drug on parturition, fertility and lactation.

   b. **Teratogenicity:** Drugs investigated on two species of animals like rat is used to test for effect on fertility, foetal organogenesis and pre- and post-natal development. The effect on development of embryo and foetus performed in rabbits.

Carcinogenicity: It detects ability of drug to induce cancers. They are performed in all drugs that are expected to be used for more than 6 months.

Phases of Clinical Trial

The clinical trial is done in four phases and each designed to address different question. The data generated from one phase is analyzed before progressing to next phase. The clinical trial studied under following phases:

1. **Phase I clinical trial:**
   a. Phase I clinical trial conducted on healthy human volunteers.
   b. Finds out drug safety in healthy human.
   c. Main purpose of initial phase I is to establish safe dosage range.
   d. Designed to determine the metabolic and pharmacological actions of the drug in human.
   e. If the drug has a potential for toxic adverse effects, it may be given only to subjects with targeted condition to reduce risk to healthy subjects (i.e. anticancer drugs are never tested in healthy volunteers).
   f. Conducted on 20–80 healthy human volunteers and typically last 3–6 months.
   g. This is a nonblind open label study.

2. **Phase II clinical trial:**
   a. Phase II clinical trial are conducted on patients.
   b. Phase II studies enroll small numbers of subjects, typically 100 to 300 and for a period of 6 month to 2 years.
   c. Main aim is to establish clinical efficacy, determine the incidence of adverse reaction, define optimum therapeutic dosage and provide detailed pharmacokinetic and pharmacological data.

3. **Phase III clinical trial:**
   a. Phase III studies are expanded controlled and uncontrolled trials.
   b. It is a multicentric trial.
   c. Performed after preliminary evidence suggesting effectiveness of the drug has been obtained.
   d. This phase involves several hundred to several thousand patients last for 1-5 years.
   e. Main aim is to establish effectiveness and adverse reaction in a large group of patients over longer periods.
   f. Phase III involve different patients subgroups, such as children, the elderly and perhaps those with impairments in liver or kidney function.
   g. Once the phase III clinical trials have been completed satisfactorily, the drug company is in a position to apply the marketing application to regulatory authorities to market the drug.

New Drug Application (NDA)

The completion of all three phases, the investigator/company analyze the data and files NDA with FDA. The regulation and control of new drugs in the United States has been based on the new drug application (NDA). Since 1938, every new drug has been the subject of an approved NDA before US commercialization. NDA is the vehicle through which drug sponsors formally propose that the FDA approved a new pharmaceutical for sale and marketing in the US. The data gathered during the animal studies and human clinical trials of an investigational new drug (IND) becomes a part of the NDA.

The goals of the NDA are to provide enough information to permit FDA reviewer to reach the following key decisions:

- Whether the drug is safe and effective in its proposed use(s), and whether the benefits of the drug outweigh the risks.
- Whether the drugs proposed labeling (package insert) is appropriate, and what it should contain.
- Whether the methods used in manufacturing the drug and the controls used to maintain the drug's quality are adequate to preserve the drug's identity, strength, quality, and purity.

The documentation required in NDA is supposed to tell the drug's whole story, including what happened during the clinical tests, what are the ingredients of the drug, the results of the animal studies, how the drug behaves in the body, and how it is manufactured, processed and packaged.

4. **Phase IV clinical trials**
    a. Phase IV clinical trials also referred as post-marketing surveillance.
    b. Sometime adverse drug reaction only come to light after the drug has been in the market for a while and has been used by a very large number of patients.

Problem Based Learning

CASE 1

A 5-years-old child is bought to the dispensary by his mother with a history of 5–6 episode of watery stool since the previous day. There is no fever, nausea or vomiting. On examination, the child pulse is higher than normal and shows sign of mild dehydration and was diagnosed to be suffering from viral diarrhoea. The mother is very anxious. What advice will you give to the mother?

Ans.

- Counsel the mother that viral diarrhoea is self-limiting condition and will subside in few days. It is viral infection and only symptomatic ℞ is required.
- Give oral rehydration solution (ORS).
- Give high carbohydrate diet like rice, khichadi, mashed potato.
- If child has developed foul smelling greenish or blood-stained stool then ask the mother to follow up with doctor.

CASE 2

A 30-years-old lady come to the gynaecology OPD with the complaints of vaginal discharge and pruritis since the past one week, per speculum examination reveals a creamy, foul smelling discharge with vascular congestion of vagina and cervix. No other abnormality is detected on vaginal examination. Wet smear of vaginal discharge demonstrates the presence of *Trichomonas vaginalis*. Your P' drug for this patient is tablet metronidazole 400 mg three times a day for 7 days. Write down the prescription for this patient. What instruction will you give to this patient?

Ans. This is a case of vaginitis due to *Trichomonas vaginalis*.

Dr ABC, MBBS   Date:.........................
Regd No: MCI123
Add: MGM Hospital
Mob No.
For
Mrs: XYZ
Age: 30   Sex: Female
Add and Mob No: Kalamboli

Tablet METRONIDAZOLE 400 mg

Dispense 21 such Tablets

One tab to be taken three times daily for 7 days

Review after 3 week

INSTRUCTION

- Male partner should be required to be prescribed the same drug.
- Follow up after 7 days for repeated smear examination.
- Avoid sexual intercourse for 7 days to prevent relapse.
- Avoid alcohol to prevent disulfiram like reaction.

Inform patient the possible side effect that is metallic test, reddish brown micturition, etc.

Refil: Nil   Doctor Sign

Generic substitution allowed   Stamp

CASE 3

An 18-years-old man present with the history of high-grade fever, severe headache, malaise, sore throat and nasal discharge since 2 days. There is no history of yellowish coloured sputum. The patient says that he took 2 tablets of Septran twice daily for one day but got no relief. On examination, he is found to have a temperature of 102°F with conjunctival and pharyngeal congestion. The patient insists on a stronger antibiotic as he says that Tab. Septran did not relive his symptoms. Your diagnosis is that of the Viral URTI. What is your therapeutic objective? Write the prescription for this patient? What advice will you give this patient?

Ans. This is case of viral URTI. As it is a self-limiting disease no antibiotics is required. A therapeutic objective is symptomatic treatment to avoid secondary infection.

Dr ABC, MBBS   Date:.....................

Regd No: MCI123

Add: MGM Hospital

Mob No.

For,

Mrs : XYZ

Age: 18   Sex: Male

Add: Kalamboli

Tablet PARACETAMOL 500 mg

Dispense 10 such Tablets

One tab to be taken three time daily till symptoms subsides
Tab CETIRIZINE 5 mg
Dispense 9 such tablets
One tab to be taken three times daily for 3 days
Review after 3 days

INSTRUCTION

- Follow up after 3–4 days.
- He should take medicine regularly.
- Warm water gargle as much as possible.
- Warn patient about sedation (ARR of Antihistamines) hence avoid driving and working with machines.

Refil: Nil   Doctor Sign

Generic substitution allowed   Stamp

CASE 4

A 40-years-old man, an occasional smoker, was diagnosed to have essential hypertension for the first time (BP 150/96 mmHg). Clinical examination revealed no other abnormality. Routine haematology and biochemical investigations as well as ECG were normal. There was no family history of hypertension. His general practitioner had prescribed Tablet Atenolol 50 mg to be taken every morning. What other advice would you like to give this patient?

Ans. This is a case of mild hypertension. The advice given to the patient is
- Avoid smoking
- Decrease salt intake
- Regular, mild exercise for long term benefit
- Avoid stress
- Regular check up
- Regular medication

CASE 5

A 19-years-old male, weighing 40 kg, presents with a history of low- grade fever, cough, anorexia and weight loss for the past two months. Sputum examination reveals the presence of acid fast bacilli. X-ray examination shows a cavitatory lesion in the right upper lobe. Your diagnosis is that of 'pulmonary tuberculosis'. What will be your therapeutic objective? What instructions will you give the patient?

Ans. Therapeutic objective is curative, i.e to clear the sputum of acid fast bacilli

INSTRUCTION

- Complete the full prescribed course.
- Prevent spread by certain precautions.
- Need for regular monitoring.
- Family members of patient may also be called for check-up.

Possible side effects should be explained like visual disturbances with Ethambutol, reddish discolouration of urine with Rifampicin, tingling and numbness with Isoniazid.

CASE 6

What precautions should be taken if a 35-year-old young male is to be given pharmacological dose of Prednisolone for a prolonged period?

Ans.

- Long term use of corticosteroids is potentially hazardous.
- Do not abruptly withdraw a corticosteroid after it has been used for than 2–3 weeks as it may precipitate adrenal insufficiency.
- Withdrawal should be done gradually by tapering the dose.
- In case of infection or trauma or stress there is marked increase in the plasma concentration of corticosteroid/glucocorticoids.
- Alternate therapy with the same glucocorticoids.

CASE 7

A 27-year-old young married lady will be prescribed Estrogen–Progesteon combination oral contraceptive pills for the next 18 months. What precautions will you take as a doctor?

Ans.

- If a lady on oral contraceptive misses a tablet she should take 2 pills the next day and then continue one pill a day as usual.
- If 2 tablet are missed the course should be stopped and mechanical barrier method of contraception should be used and next course should be started from 5th day of menstruation as usual.
- If pregnancy occurs during the use of oral contraceptive use, it should be terminated due to risk of genital carcinoma in female offsprings or undescended testis in male.

CASE 8

Mrs Balkrishan was suffering from grandmal epilepsy. She was getting Phenobarbitone 80 mg daily. Her fits were well controlled. Since her child was just one year old, she started taking oral contraceptive. But to her surprise, she became pregnant.

   a. What do you think is the cause of failure of oral contraceptive therapy? (non-complaince by the patient was ruled out)
   b. If the patient continues phenobarbitone, what alternative would you suggest for contraception?

Ans.

- As Phenobarbitone is a microsomal enzyme inducer, it metabolises the oral contraceptive and reduces its therapeutic effect.
- If she continues Phenobarbitone alternative method of contraception should be used.

CASE 9

Mr. Murli Mohan aged 30-years is suffering from amoebiasis for which he is under treatment. After few drinks in cocktail party, he felt sick with palpitation and marked flushing.

a. What could be the cause of the sickness?

b. What instruction the treating physician should have given to the patient?

Ans.

- He developed Disulfiram like reaction.
- He is adviced to avoid alcohol during treatment on Metronidazole.

CASE 10

A 55-years-old lady was on Propranolol treatment for hypertension and her blood pressure was under control. She went to dentist for tooth extraction. The dentist gave Xylocaine with adrenaline for local anesthesia. The patient's blood pressure shot up to 190/100 mm of Hg and pulse rate went down to 40/min.

a. Explain the mechanism of complication?

b. How will you treat this case?

Ans.

- Propranolol is β blocker which blocks β_2 receptor on blood vessels. When Xylocaine was given with adrenaline it raises the blood pressure significantly by acting on the vasoconstrictory α receptor on blood vessels since the vasodilator β_2 were blocked. Hence there was rise in BP.
- This can be treated by giving only Xylocaine and avoiding its combination with adrenaline.

CASE 11

Mr Sundar who is on Chlorpromazine therapy for schizophrenia developed Parkinsonism. He was prescribed L-dopa 250 mg 4 times a day. He was not relieved, so the dose of L-dopa was increased to 750 mg 4 times a day. Even then he was not benefited.

a. What could be the reason?

b. Will you suggest any other drug for the control of Parkinsonism?

Ans.

- Drug induced parkinsonism as D2 receptors are blocked by Chlorpromazine. Therefore L-dopa will not produce any beneficial effect in Parkinsonism.
- Anticholinergic drugs can be used as alternative drug.

CASE 12

A diabetic patient is stabilized on diet and insulin. He is prescribed Prednisolone 10 mg daily for joint pains.

a. Will it have any effect on his diabetic state?

b. Will you consider any change in the treatment?

Ans.

- Prednisolone being a corticosteroid may aggravate his diabetic condition.
- Alternative drug like NSAIDS should be given.

CASE 13

A child aged 1 year comes with watery diarrhoea was given tab Loperamide. Comment on therapy.

Ans. Loperamide should not be used in children below 4 year of age because paralytic ileus, toxic megacolon with abdominal distention is a serious complication in young children. Fatalities have occurred probably due to absorption of toxins from intestine.

CASE 14

In a suspected case of morphine poisoning, 5 mg of Nalorphine was given IV by a doctor.

a. Comment on the choice of antidote.

Ans. Naloxone IV is the drug of choice as an antidote for Morphine poisoning. Naloxone is a competitive μ opioid-receptor antagonist that reverses all signs of opioid intoxication. On the other hand, Nalorphine is a mixed opioid agonist-antagonist with opioid antagonist and analgesic properties. Therefore the pure opioid antagonist Naloxone is preferred over Nalorphine as a choice of antidote for Morphine poisoning.

CASE 15

A 2-year-old child was taken to the dentist for the treatment of caries. The dentist noticed brownish-yellow discoloration of teeth. On inquiring, mother of the child said that she had not received any antibiotic other than penicillin and during her pregnancy, she was treated for trachoma with some capsules.

a. What is the cause of brownish-yellow discoloration of child's teeth?

b. Could it have been prevented?

Ans. The mother must have been treated with tetracycline for trachoma. Tetracylines are known to cause brownish-yellow discoloration of teeth. Tooth staining/ discoloration with tetracycline is influenced by the dosage used, length of treatment or exposure, stage of tooth mineralization and degree of activity of the mineralization process. The discoloration is permanent and can vary from yellow or gray to brown.Tetracycline can cause staining if taken anytime from the second trimester of pregnancy to 12 years of age by bonding with the calcium ions in the body. Calcium ions acquire during tooth development, and the stain becomes part of the tooth structure. Yes, it could have been prevented, if tetracycline was avoided during pregnancy.

Criticism on Prescription

How do you criticise a given prescription?

Any answer to a question on criticism always contains two parts:

A. Actual criticism of the prescription
   - The prescription must be complete in its format.
   - Details prescribed therapy.
   - Check the completeness of the prescribing information like dosage form, generic name, strength, amount, frequency, duration.
   - Select correct drugs, if not then justfy your reasons for not prescribing the same.
   - Mention why the drug is contraindicated/harmful in the given situation, i.e. whether it may your reasons for not prescribing the same.
   - Check if any non pharmacological therapy has been advised, if not, then make the necessary observation on the same, making sure to be specific and giving quantities, wherever so advised.

B. Rewriting of the correct prescription
   - When doing this, ensure the prescription is in a proper format.
   - Prescribe all the indicated drug therapy; include proper and specific non-pharmacological therapy whenever needed.
   - Do not use any abbreviation, unless universally accepted.
   - Rewrite prescription with your criticism.

1. Comment, correct and rewrite the following prescription for a patient of insulin dependent diabetes mellitus with mild hypertension.

Dr. ABC
MBBS
Regd. No. MCI 44700
Kharghar, Mumbai
Mob No:

For

Mr. Leonard Thompson

1. Inj. Lente insulin 40 units IM TDs
2. Tab Propranolol 40 mg TDs

Criticism

- Prescription is not in a proper format.
- **Lente insulin:** Indication and dose is right. Frequency of administration is wrong, because lente insulin is intermediate acting insulin preparation, it can be given twice a day. Route of administration is wrong, because insulin should be given subcutaneously for uniform and sustained effect in this case.

  Insulin is absolutely essential for the patient of insulin dependent diabetes mellitus. It decreases blood sugar level by stimulating the uptake, utilization and storage of glucose and inhibiting glucose production by glycogenolysis and neoglucogenesis. It also corrects the metabolic disorders and prevents the complications of diabetes mellitus. Readymade mixtures of actrapid and purified NPH insulin (Mixtard) should be used as onset of action of lente insulin is two hours.
- **Propranolol:** Indication is wrong. Propranolol is contraindicated in a patient of IDDM, as it is non-selective β-blocker. Because, it may delay the recovery from insulin-induced hypoglycemia by blocking β_2 receptors in the liver which mediate glycogenolysis. In addition to blocking glycogenolysis, propranolol can interfere with the perception of symptoms such as tremors, tachycardia and nervousness. ACE-inhibitor such as enalapril is the anti-hypertensive of choice in patient of IDDM, as it delays diabetic nephropathy.

Corrected prescription:

Name: Dr. ABC; MBBS, MD (Medicine)	Date: 12/10/2020

Regd no: MCI 125
Addres: Kharghar
Mob No:
Patient name: Mr Leonard thompson
Age: 40
Gender: Male
Body weight: 55 kg
Address and Contact No: Kharghar

Injection MIXTARD 10 ml vial (40 units/ml)
Send one such vial.
One ml to be injected subcutaneously 30 min. before breakfast and 30 min before dinner daily.
Tablet ENALAPRIL 5 mg
Send 7 such tablets
One tablet to be taken in the morning daily.
Follow up after one week.
Refil: Nil　　　　　　　　　　　　　　　　　　　　Doctor Sign
Generic substitution allowed　　　　　　　　　　　　Stamp

2. Comment, correct and rewrite the following prescription for a patient of congestive cardiac failure.

Dr. ABC
MBBS
Regd. No. 44700

For
Mrs Aparna V. Jogalekar
Age: 49 years

1. Tab Digoxin 0.25 mg OD
2. Tab Furosemide 40 mg OD

Criticism

- Prescription is not in a proper format.
- **Digoxin:** Indication, dose, frequency of administration and route is correct. In congestive cardiac failure, heart is not able to maintain the normal cardiac output required for the body. Digoxin is a positive inotropic drug. It increases force of contraction of heat. It does not increase heart rate. It increases cardiac output by increasing the stroke volume with less oxygen consumption.
- **Furosemide:** Indication is wrong. Furosemide is used in severe case of congestive cardiac failure, which is not responding to Thiazide diuretic. It should not be used in mild to moderate case of congestive cardiac failure, as it produces many adverse effects.

Corrected prescription:

Name: Dr. ABC; MBBS, MD (Medicine)   Date: 5/5/2020
Regd no: MCI 125
Addres: Kharghar
Mob No:
Patient name: Mrs Aparna
Age: 49
Gender: Female
Weight: 50 kg
Address and Contact No: Kharghar

Tablet DIGOXIN 0.25 mg
Send 5 such tablets
One tablet is to be taken daily
Tablet HYDROCHLOROTHIAZIDE 25 mg
Send 7 such tablets.
One tablet is to be taken daily in the morning on empty stomach.
Syrup POTASSIUM CHLORIDE 5 mmol/ml, 100 ml bottle
Send 1 such bottle.
5 ml diluted in a glass of water to be given orally two times daily.
Review after 1 week
Refil: Nil   Doctor sign
Generic substitution allowed   Stamp

3. Comment, correct and rewrite the following prescription for a 9 year child suffering from fever.

Dr. ABC
MBBS
Regd. No. 44700
Dadar west
Mumbai
Date:

For
Mr. Rohan D. Athawale
Sex: Male Age: 9 years
Address: 61, Katepuram,
Mumbai

Tab Aspirin 300 mg ½ TDs

Criticism

- Prescription is not in a proper format.
- **Aspirin:** Indication is wrong. Aspirin is contraindicated in children with fever. Because, the cause of fever could be viral such as influenza or varicella. Aspirin can cause Rey's syndrome if given in presence of viral fever in children. Rey's syndrome is characterized by hepatic damage and encephalopathy. This has serious and often fatal complication.

Corrected prescription:

Name: Dr. ABC; MBBS, MD (Medicine) Regd no: MCI 125 Addres: Kharghar Mob No: Patient name: Mr. Rohan Age: 9 Gender: Male Weight: 25 kg Address and contact No: 61, Kate puram, Mumbai	Date: 12/12/2020

℞

Tablet PARACETAMOL 500 mg
Send 5 such tablets.
½ tablet to be given thrice a day.
Review after 3 days
Refil: Nil
Generic substitution allowed

Doctor sign
Stamp

4. Comment, correct and rewrite the following prescription for a patient of drug-induced parkinsonism.

Dr. ABC
MBBS
Regd. No. 44700

For
Mr. Santosh Meshram
Sex: Male, Age: 37 years

Inj. Diazepam 5 mg IM

Dr. S. M. Khan

Criticism

- Prescription is not in a proper format.
- Diazepam: Indication is wrong. Diazepam can be used in drug-induced parkinsonism as it produces skeletal muscle relaxation. But it is not the drug of choice. Centrally acting anticholinergic drug such as benzhexol should be used for this condition. Because, usually it is caused by hyperactivity of central cholinergic system.

Corrected prescription:

Name: Dr. ABC; MBBS, MD (Medicine)	Date: 2/2/2020

Regd no: MCI 125
Addres: Kharghar
Mob No:
Patient name: Mr. Santosh Meshram
Age: 37
Gender: Male
Weight: 65 kg
Address and Contact No: 61, Kate puram

Tablet BENZHEXOL 2 mg
Send 7 such tablets
One tablet is to be taken once daily.
Review after 7 days

Refil: Nil

Generic substitution allowed

Doctor sign

Stamp

5. Comment, correct and rewrite the following prescription for a patient of deep vein thrombosis with backache.

Dr. ABC
MBBS
Regd. No. 44700
Dadar west

For
Mrs. Manisha V. Shirsat
Sex: Female, Age: 35 years
Address: 13, Vaishalinagar

1. Tab Warfarin sodium 5 mg OD
2. Tab Aspirin 600 mg 2 TDs

Criticism

- Prescription is not in proper format.
- **Warfarin sodium:** Indication, dose, frequency of administration and route is correct. Warfarin sodium is an oral anticoagulant which is used in deep vein thrombosis.
- **Aspirin:** Indication is wrong. Aspirin in large dose reduce the plasma prothrombin level by interfering with the action of vitamin K in the liver. Aspirin produces synergistic effect with warfarin on prothrombin synthesis. Hence, aspirin in large dose should be avoided in this patient.

Corrected prescription:

Name: Dr. ABC; MBBS, MD (Medicine) Regd no: MCI 125 Addres: Kharghar Mob No:	Date: 12/10/2020

Name: Mrs. Manisha V. Shirsat
Age: 35
Gender: Female
Weight: 45 kg
Address and Contact No: 13, Vaishalinagar, Mumbai

Rx

Tablet WARFARIN SODIUM 5 mg
Send 7 such tablets
One tablet is to be taken once daily.
Tablet PARACETAMOL 500 mg
Send 15 such tablets
One tablet is to be taken three times a day.
Review after 1 week
Refil: Nil

Doctor sign
Stamp

Generic substitution allowed

6. Comment, correct and rewrite the following prescription for a patient of peptic ulcer.

Dr. ABC
MBBS

Tab Cimetidine 200 mg OD
Cap Omeprazole 40 mg TD
Cap Sucralfate 1 g OD
Liq. Aluminium hydroxide gel 10 ml OD

Criticism

- Prescription is not in a proper format.
- **Cimetidine:** Indication, dose, frequency of administration and route is correct, it is histamine H_2 receptor blocker used in peptic ulcer to reduce acid secretion. However, it produces more adverse effects related to antiandrogenic actions and inhibition of drug metabolizing enzymes in the liver. Other H_2 blockers such as Ranitidine or Famotidine are preferred, as they have less adverse effects, selective and longer duration of action. Within 2 hours of its administration Sucralfate or Aluminium hydroxide should not be given, as they decrease its bioavailability. It is not necessary to combine it with Omeprazole which is also antisecretory.
- **Omeprazole:** Indication, and route is correct, but it is not necessary to combine with H_2 blocker. Frequency of administration is wrong, it is once a day.
- **Sucralfate:** Indication, Dose and route is correct, but it should not be given with antacid. Frequency of administration is wrong, it is 3 to 4 times a day.
- **Liq. Aluminium hydroxide gel:** Indication and dose is correct, but it should not be given with H_2 blockers or Sucralfate. Dose: 10 ml at 1 hour and 3 hours after each meal

Corrected prescription:

Name: Dr. ABC; MBBS, MD (Medicine)	Date: 12/12/2020
Regd no: MCI 125	
Addres: Kharghar	
Mob No:	
Name: Mr. Tushar B. Gangane	
Age: 35	
Gender: Male	
Weight: 48 kg	
Address and Contact No.: 13, Vaishalinagar, Mumbai	

Capsule OMEPRAZOLE 20 mg
Send 10 such capsules
One capsule to be taken in the morning.
Follow up after 1 week.
Refil: Nil   Doctor sign
Generic substitution allowed   Stamp

7. Comment, correct and rewrite the following prescription for a patient of UTI during pregnancy.

Dr. ABC
MBBS
Regd. No. 44700
Dadar west
Mumbai
Date:

For
Mrs Jyoti V. Howale
Sex: Female   Age: 31 years
Address: 61, Kate puram
Mumbai

Tab Cotrimoxazole 1 BID for 5 days

Criticism

* Prescription is not in proper format.
* **Cotrimoxazole:** Indication is wrong, it is contraindicated in pregnancy. Cotrimoxazole is fixed drug combination which contains Sulfamethoxazole 400 mg + Trimethoprim 80 mg. Trimethoprim in large doses is reported to be teratogenic in animals. So, it should be avoided during pregnancy.

Corrected prescription:

Name: Dr. ABC; MBBS, MD (Medicine)   Date: 10/10/2020
Regd no: MCI 125
Addres: Kharghar
Mob No:
Name: Mrs Jyoti V Howale
Age: 31
Gender: Female
Weight: 60 kg
Address and Contact No: 61, Kate puram, Mumbai
℞
Capsule AMOXICILLIN 500 mg
Send 21 such capsules
One capsule to be taken thrice a day
Review after 1 week
Refil: Nil   Doctor sign
Generic substitution allowed   Stamp

Skill Assessment on Mannequin: Administration of Medication by Various Route (DOAP)

How to apply Topical Medication

1. Wash the affected area(s) of skin well and rinse away all traces of soap or cleanser. Pat the skin dry rather than rubbing it.
2. Apply the cream or ointment thinly and evenly to the affected area(s).
3. Gently massage the cream or ointment into the skin until it has all disappeared.
4. If you have other creams, ointments or lotions to use on the same area of skin you should try and leave about half an hour between applying each one so that they don't mix on the skin.

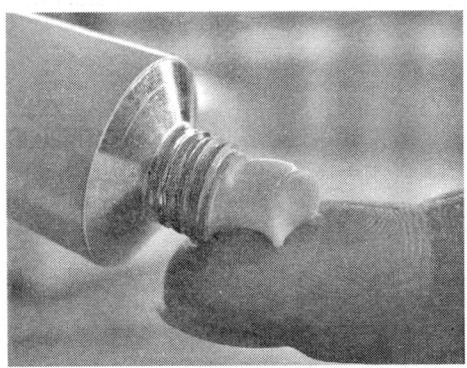 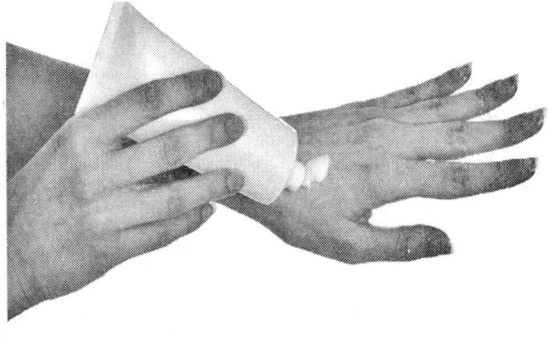

Fig. 12.1

How to Instill Ophthalmic Medication

1. Hold filled medications, eye dropper or ophthalmic solution approximately 1–2 cm above conjunctival sac.
2. **For instilling eye drop:** Pull the lower lid down to expose the conjunctival sac. Have the patients look up and away, then squeeze the prescribed number of drops into the sac. Release the patients eyelid and have him/her to rotate the age ball distribute the medication.
3. If drop land on outer lid margin, repeat procedure.
4. **For instilling eye ointment:** Gently lay a thin strip of the medication along the conjunctival sac from the inner canthus to the outer canthus and avoid touching

the tips of the tube to the patients eye. Then release the eye lid and have the patients roll his/her eye behind closed lids to distribute the medication.

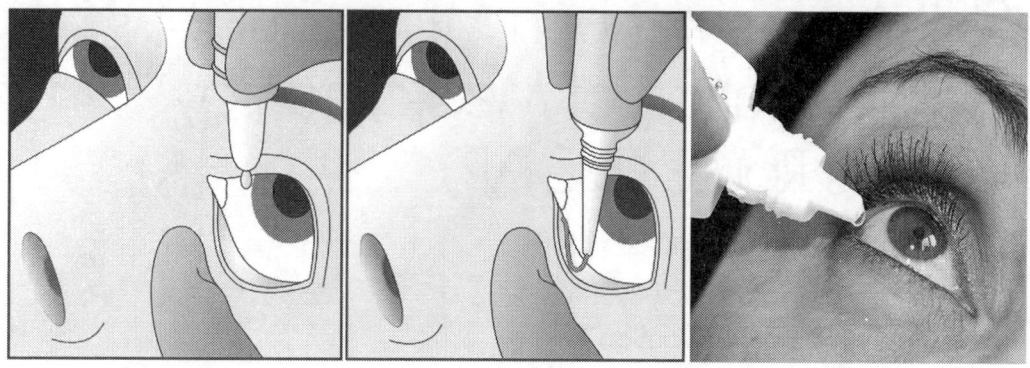

| Eye drops | Eye ointment |

Fig. 12.2

How to Instill Otic Medication

1. Wash your hands with soap and water.
2. Before instilling eardrops, allow the patients lie on his or her side.
3. Hold filled medication dropper approximately 1–2 cm above ear canal.
4. Then straighten the ear canal to help the medication reach the eardrum.
5. For adult, gently pull the auricle up and back.
6. For young child and infant gently pull down and back.

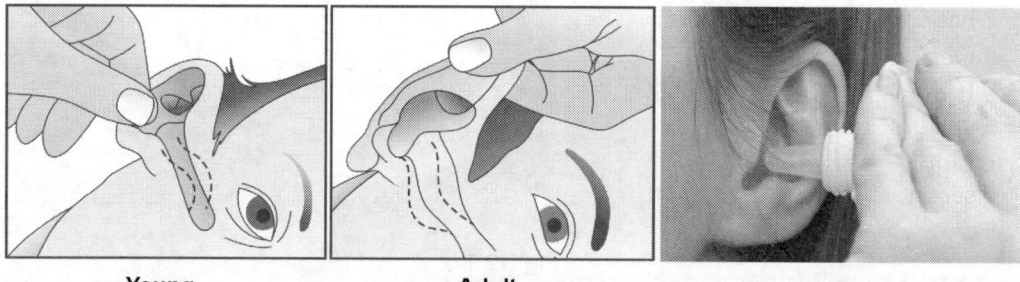

| Young | Adult |

Fig. 12.3

How to Instill Nasal Medication

1. Wash your hands thoroughly with soap and water.
2. Gently blow your nose to clear your nasal passages.
3. Avoid touching the dropper tip against your clean nose.
4. Tilt your head as far back as possible, or lie down on your back on a flat surface.
5. Place the correct number of drops into your nose.
6. Bend your head forward toward your knees and gently move it left and right.
7. Remain in this position for a few minutes.

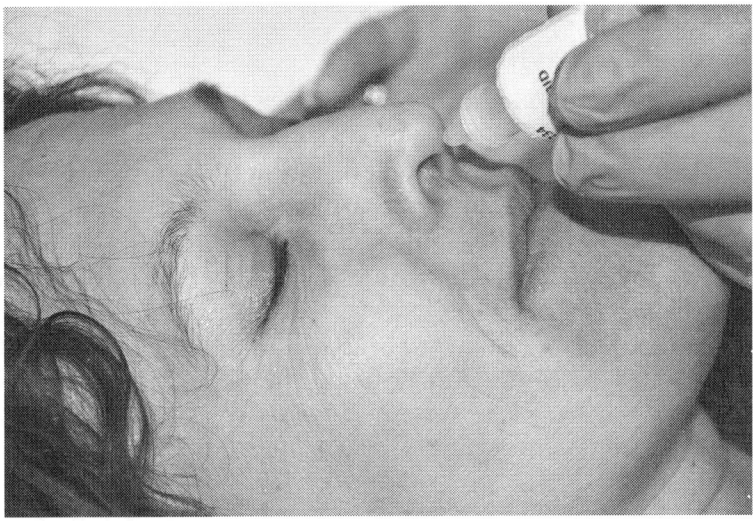

Fig. 12.4

How to Take Oral medicine

The most common way people take medications is orally (by mouth). Depending on what your physician prescribed, oral medication can be swallowed, chewed, or placed under your tongue to dissolve.

1. Wash hands with soap and warm water.
2. Assist patients to an upright or lateral position.
3. Open any pre-packaged medications and place the tablets/capsule in the patients hand, provide adequate amount of water.
4. Observe the patients until all medication is safely swallowed.
5. If tablet are dissolvable or dispersible, ensure the entire volume of solution is swallowed.
6. Liquid oral medications will require gentle shaking of the medication for a few seconds to ensure the equal distribution of the medication within the liquid.

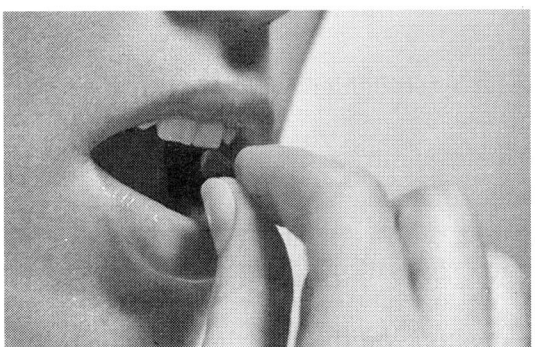 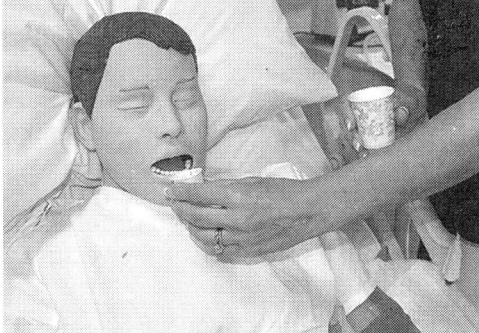

Fig. 12.5

How to Take Sublingual/Buccal Medicine

1. Wash hands with soap and warm water.
2. Open any pre-packaged medications and place the medication in the patient's hand.
3. The person taking sublingual or buccal medication should always be situated in an upright position before administration of medicaments.
4. Do not allow the individual to lie down or try to administer the medication when the person is unconscious. This could, lead to accidental aspiration of the medication.
5. To give a drug buccally, insert it between the patients cheek and gum. Tell patient to close his mouth and hold the tablet against his cheek until it absorbed.
6. To give a drug sublingually, put it under the patients tongue and ask to leave it there until dissolved.

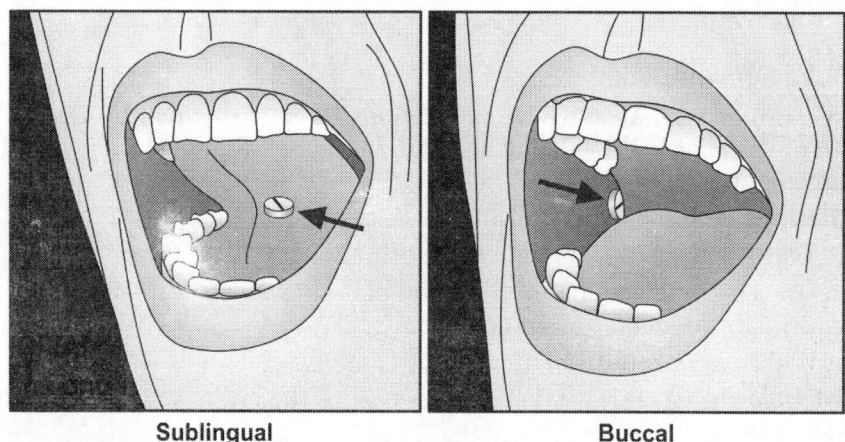

| Sublingual | Buccal |

Fig. 12.6

How to Use Rectal Medicine

1. Wash your hands thoroughly with soap and hot water.
2. Put on a finger cot or disposable glove.
3. Patients should be lying on side with lower leg straightened out and upper leg bent forward toward stomach.
4. Hold one buttock gently to one side so that you can see the rectum.
5. Unwrap the medicine and hold it with the rounded end close to the rectum.
6. Insert the suppository, rounded end first, with your finger until it passes the muscular sphincter of the rectum, about 1/2 to 1 inch in infants and 1 inch in adults.
7. Remain lying down for about 5 minutes to avoid having the medicine come out.

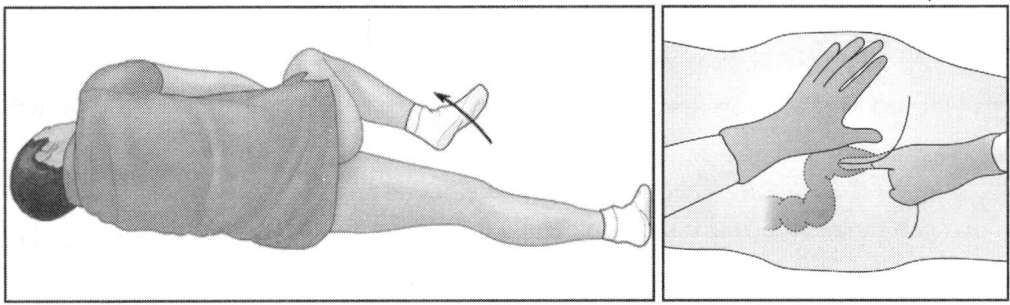

Fig. 12.7

Injections

It is an infusion method of putting fluid into the body, usually with a syringe and a hollow needle which is pierced through the skin to a sufficient depth for the material to be administered into the body.

Syringe is a device made of a hollow tube and a needle that is used to force fluids into or take fluids out of the body.

Parts of Syringe

Three main parts of syringe

1. **Barrel:** Chamber that holds the medication.
2. **Plunger:** Part within the barrel that moves back and forth to withdraw and instill medication.
3. **Tip:** Part that the needle is attached.

Needles: Shaft of the needle length chosen depends on the depth to which medication will be instilled. Tip of shaft is beveled or slanted to pierce the skin more easily.
Gauge: Width of the needle (18–27 gauge). A smaller number indicates a larger diameter and larger lumen inside the needle.

The correct needle is the key to delivering the drug to the correct area for the maximum effect with the least amount of discomfort. The colour at the top of the needle reflects its size, the higher the number the smaller the lumen (bore).

Orange needles = 25 gauge = 10 mm long (3/8 inch) or 16 mm long (5/8 inch) or 25 mm long (1 inch).

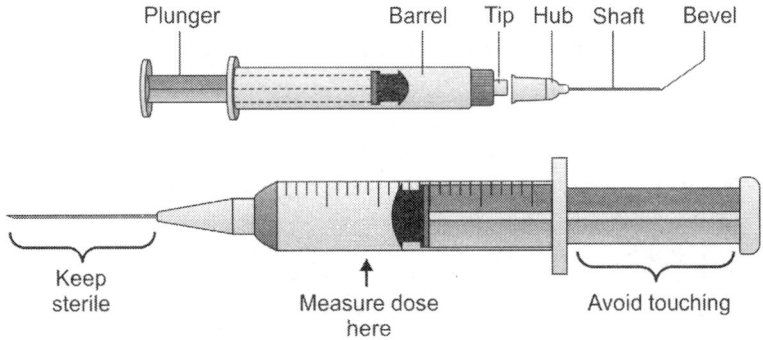

Fig. 12.8

Blue needles = 23 gauge = 25 mm long (1 inch)
Green needles = 21 gauge = 38 mm long (1.5 inches)

Drawing up Medication from a Ampoule

1. Wash hands and grasp the stem with an alcohol swab.
2. Snap off the ampoules neck away from the hands and face.
3. Uncap the needle and insert the needle into the ampoule avoid touching the rim with the needle.
4. Invert the ampoule, insert the needle into the solution and aspirate.
5. Remove the needle cap and draw an amount of air into the syringe that is equal to the amount of medication that will be withdrawn from the ampoule.

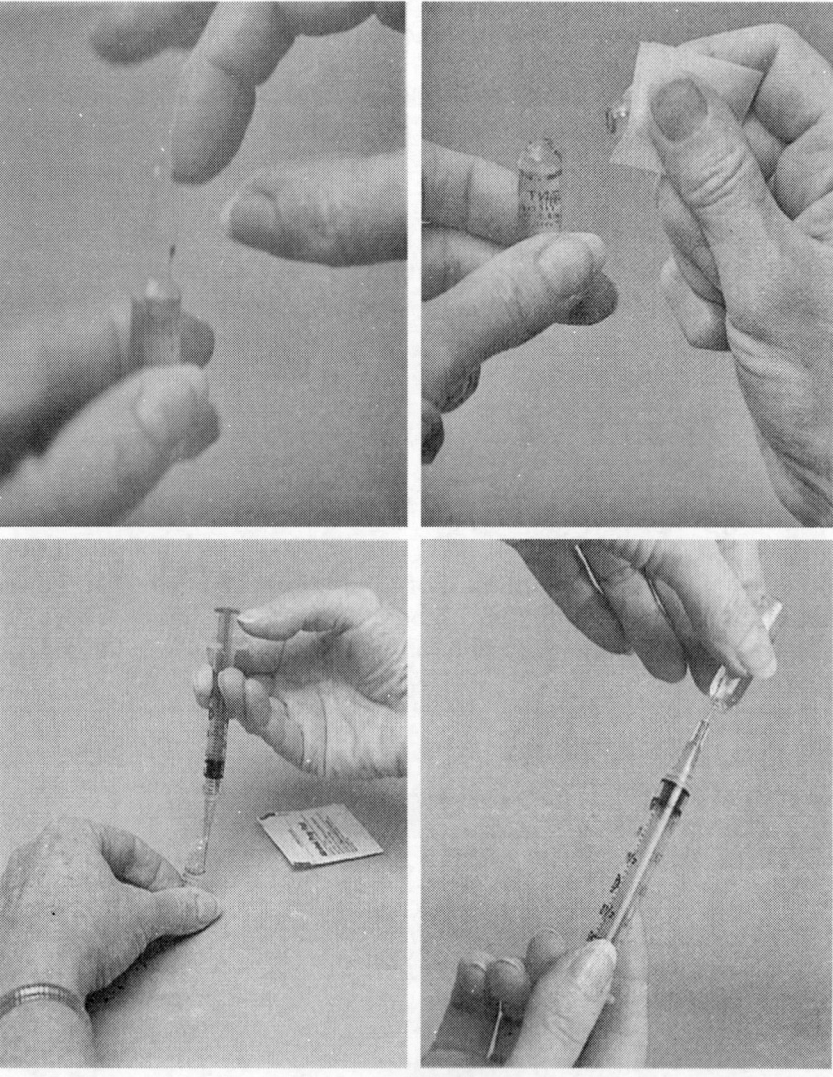

Fig. 12.9

Drawing Up Medication from a Vial

1. Wash hands and insert the needle keeping it above the solution.
2. Invert the vial at eye level.
3. Hold the needle upright and re-check the syringe content for presence of air.

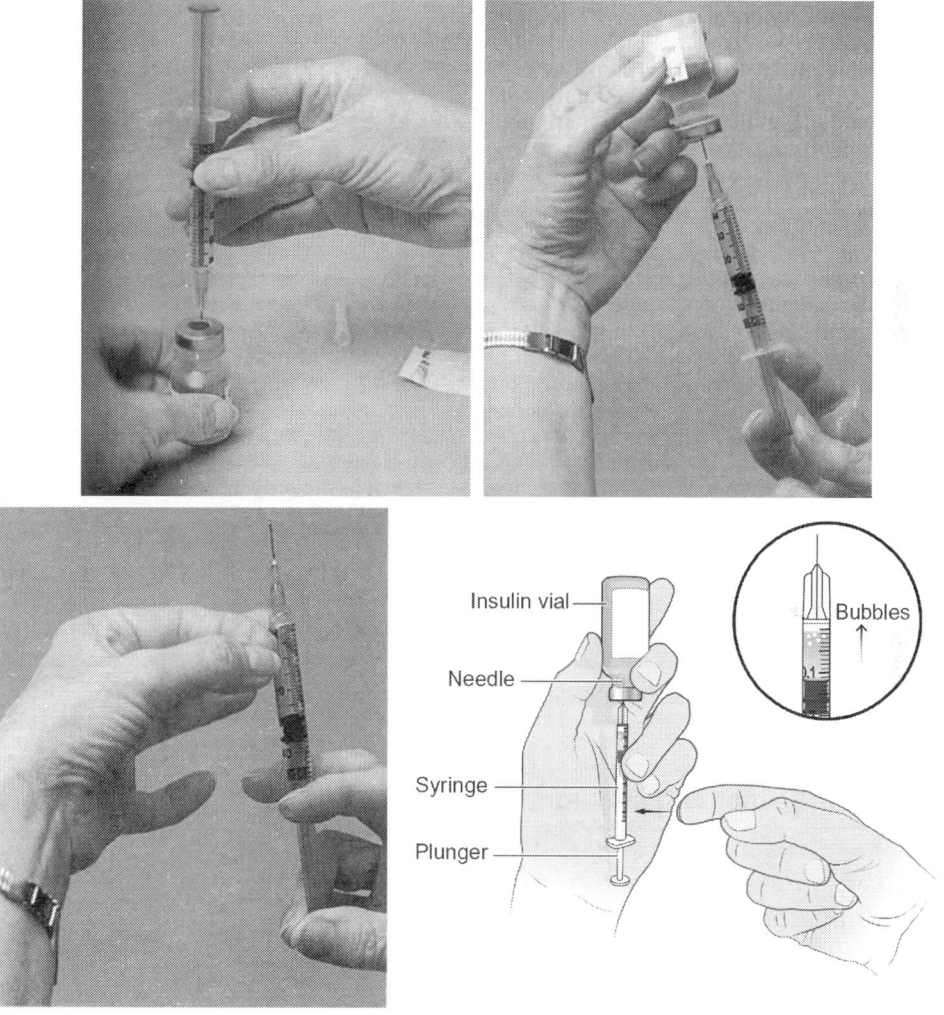

Fig. 12.10: Showing of drawing up medication from a vial

How to Give Injection by Intradermal Route

1. The injection site is rubbed vigorously with a swab and disinfectant applied to cleanse the area and increase the blood supply.
2. Support skin with thumb with bevel up, completely insert bevel at a 15 degree angle.

3. Intradermal injections are usually given on the inner surface of the forearm. With the bevel of the needle facing upwards at 15° angle, the needle is inserted into the skin, parallel to the forearm. The syringe should then be pushed-in steadily and slowly, releasing the solution into the layers of the skin. This will cause the layers of skin to rise slightly.

4. Since intradermal injections do not involve the penetration of major blood vessels, you do not need to aspirate the syringe.

5. If a wheal, or bleb, does not appear during administration, the medication is being delivered into the subcutaneous tissue.

6. Dispose of needle as per policy.

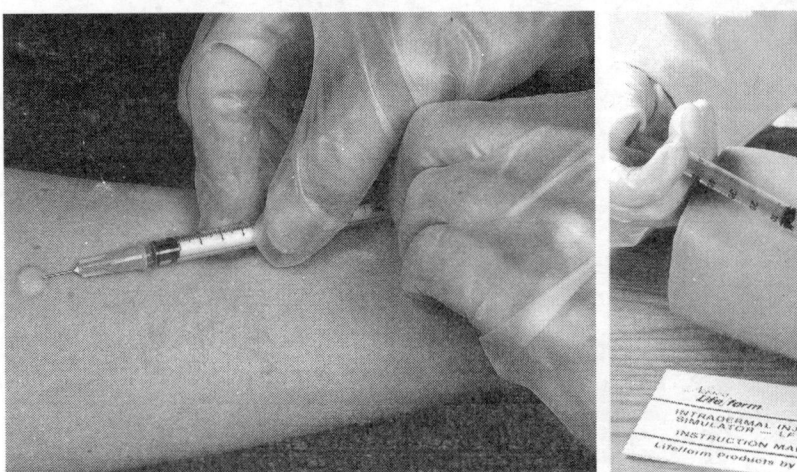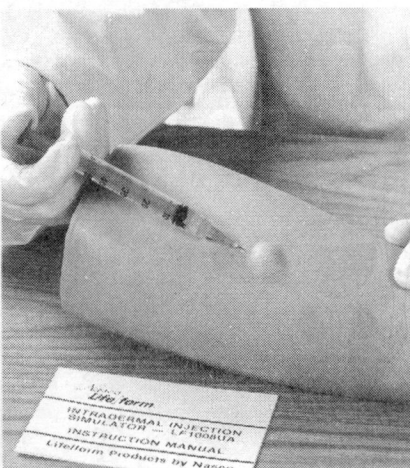

Fig. 12.11: Showing intradermal injection technique

How to Give Injection by Subcutaneous Route

1. Common sites used for subcutaneous route are outer aspect of the upper arm, abdomen (from below the costal margin to the iliac crests), anterior aspects of the thigh, upper back, upper ventral or dorsogluteal area.

2. Apply swap and rotated outwards in circular direction. Hold syringe in the dominant hand between the thumb and forefinger.

3. Take a big pinch of skin between your thumb and index finger and hold it (your thumb and forefinger should be about an inch and a half apart). This pulls the fatty tissue away from the muscle and makes the injection easier.

4. Inject the needle quickly at an angle of 45 to 90 degree, depending on the amount and turgor of the tissue and the length of the needle.

5. Dispose of needle as per policy.

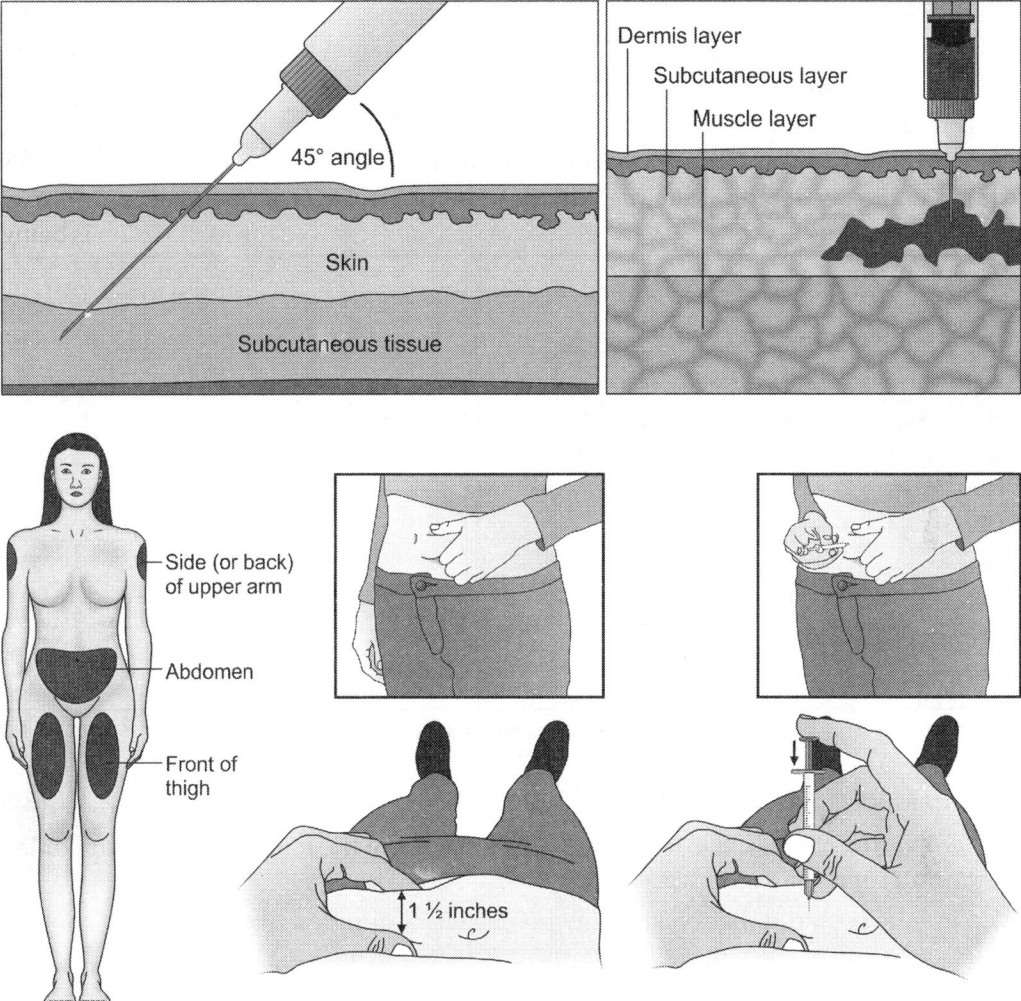

Fig. 12.12: Showing subcutaneous injection technique

How to give Injection by Intramuscular Route

1. Clean the site selected for injection with an alcohol swab and allow the skin to air dry.

2. Insert the needle into the muscle at a 90 degree angle. Use the index finger and thumb to stabilize the syringe while using the other hand to pull back on the plunger slightly to look for blood.

3. If there is blood, it means the needle is in a blood vessel and not in muscle. Withdraw and start over with a new needle, syringe and injection site. If there is no blood, the needle is in the correct position. Press down on the plunger of the syringe to inject the medication.

4. Dispose of needle as per policy.

Deltoid Site

1. Find the knobbly top of the arm (acromion process).
2. The top border of an inverted triangle is two finger widths down from the acromion process.
3. Stretch the skin and then bunch up the muscle.
4. Insert the needle at a right angle to the skin in the centre of the inverted triangle.

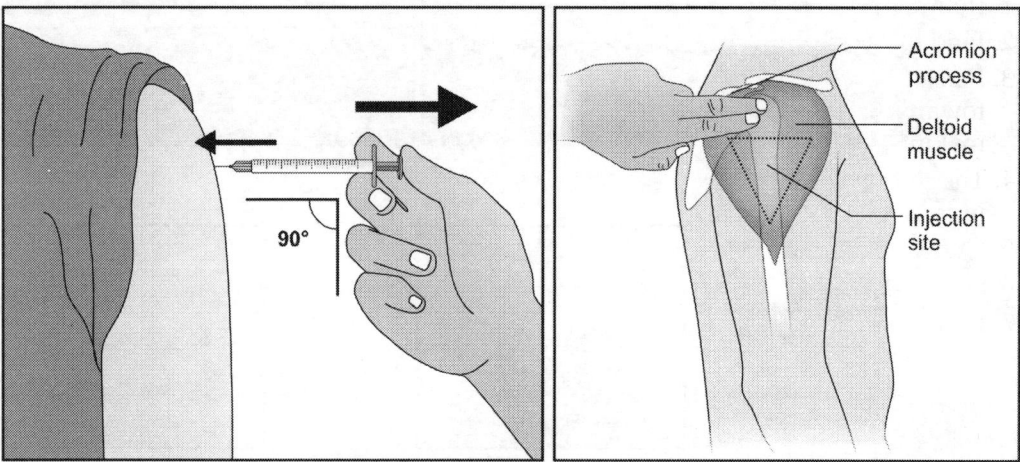

Fig. 12.13: Showing injection technique in deltoid site

Gluteus Medius Site (Buttock)

1. Find the trochanter. It is the knobbly top portion of the long bone in the upper leg (femur). It is the size of a golf ball.
2. Find the posterior iliac crest. Many people have 'dimples' over this bone.
3. Draw an imaginary line between the two bones.

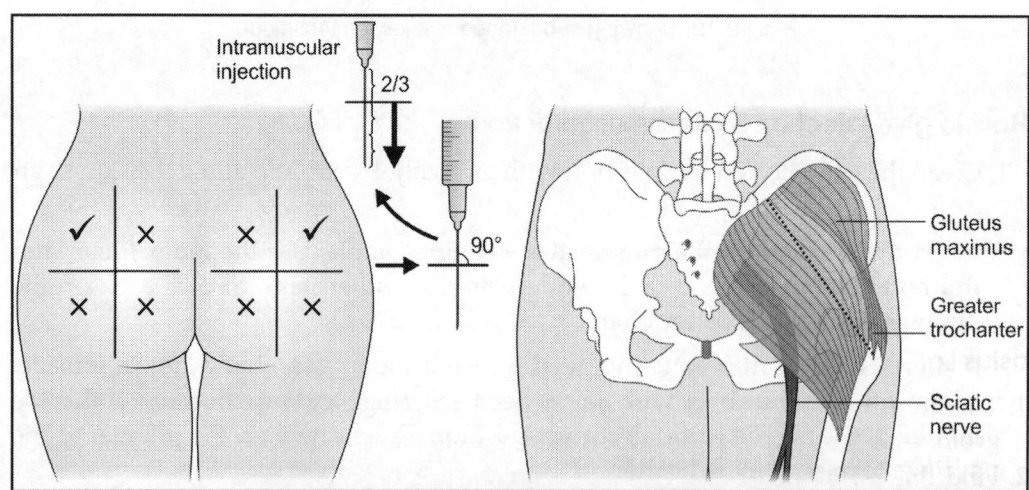

Fig. 12.14: Showing injection technique in gluteus medius site

4. After locating the centre of the imaginary line, find a point one inch toward the head. This is where (√) to insert the needle.
5. Stretch the skin tight.
6. Hold the syringe like a pencil. Insert the needle at a right angle into the muscle.

Ventrogluteal Site

1. Find the trochanter. It is the knobbly top portion of the long bone in the upper leg (femur). It is about the size of a golf ball.
2. Find the anterior iliac crest.
3. Place the palm of your hand over the trochanter. Point the first or index finger toward the anterior iliac crest. Spread the second or middle finger toward the back, making a 'V'.
4. The thumb should always be pointed toward the front of the leg. Always use the index finger and middle finger to make the 'V'.
5. Give the injection between the knuckles on your index and middle fingers.
6. Stretch the skin tight.
7. Hold the syringe like a pencil or dart. Insert the needle at a right angle to the skin (90°).

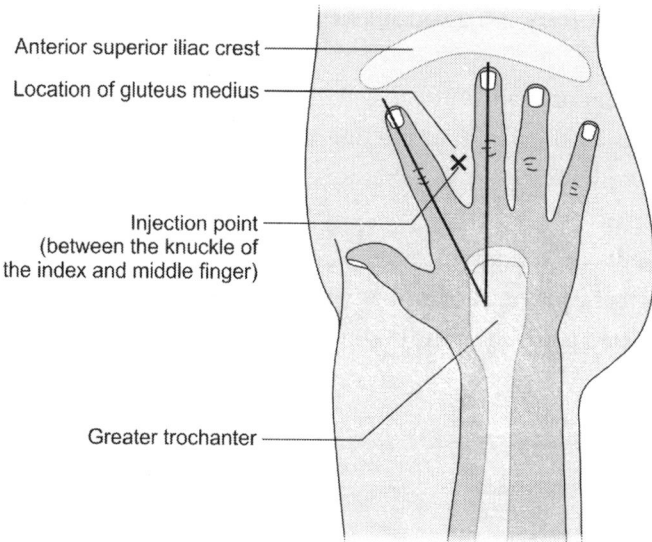

Fig. 12.15: Showing injection technique in ventrogluteal site

Vastus Lateralis Site

1. To find the thigh injection site, make an imaginary box on the upper leg. Find the groin. One hand's width below the groin becomes the upper border of the box.
2. Find the top of knee. One hand's width above the top of the knee becomes the lower border of the box.

3. Stretch the skin to make it tight.
4. Insert the needle at a right angle to the skin (90°) straight.

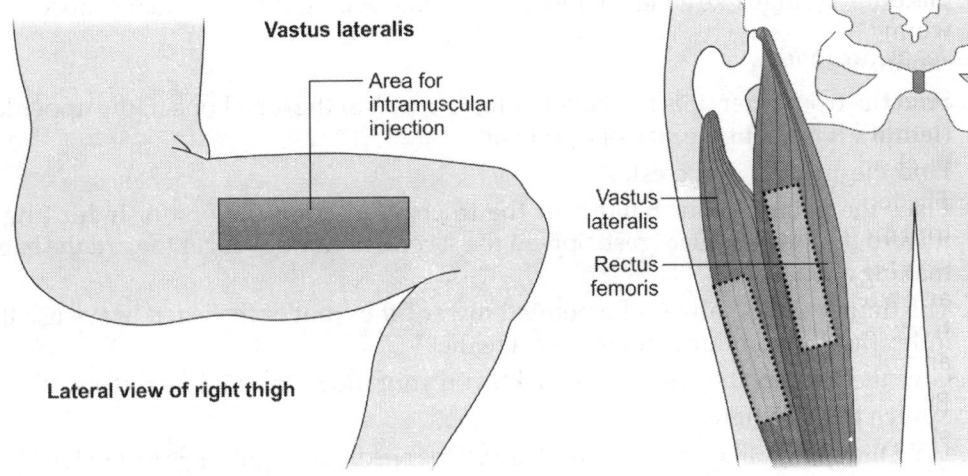

Fig. 12.16: Showing injection technique in vastus lateralis site

How to Give Injection by Intravenous Route in Arm

Procedure

1. Apply tourniquet on arm.
2. Choose median basilica vein or medial cephalic vein.
3. Palpitate the vein.
4. Apply antiseptic.
5. Insert the needle at 30 degree angle.
6. Release the tourniquet and complete the injection.
7. Apply sterile pad prior to withdrawal of syringe.

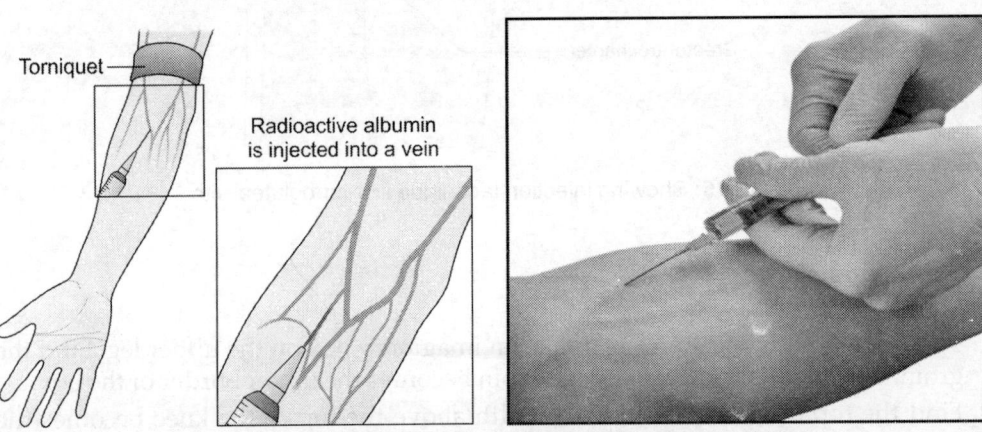

Fig. 12.17: Showing intravenous injection technique

How to Insert IV Cannula

Procedure

1. When choosing an appropriate vein for venipuncture, a cannula should not be placed in area of localized oedema, dermatitis, cellulitis, arteriovenous fistulae, wounds, skin grafts, fractures, stroke, planned limb surgery and site of previous cannulation.
2. Select a vein, if the site is excessively hairy, the hair should be clipped, the site should not be shaved because it causes micro abrasions. Visibly dirty skin should be cleaned with soap and water.
3. The tourniquet is applied 2–3 inches above the intended venipuncture site, when tourniquet is in place, the patient should be asked to open and dose his fist several times to encourage venous distension. Gently rubbing or stroking the arm to warm the skin, and covering the entire arm with moist compresses also triggers the vasodilation. The vein should be palpated gently to see if it feels soft and bouncy.
4. Before performing venipuncture, the vein should be stretched and immobilized steps.
5. The right hand should be used to grasp the cannula or the cannulas wings and proceed at once with venipuncture.
6. The cannula should be inserted at 30 degree angle bevel upwards.
7. The blood backflow in the cannula tubing or hub should be observed as it signifies that the cannula is in the vein lumen.
8. Once the backflow has been observed, the cannula is lowered almost parallel to skin. The catheter is then pushed off the stellate and advanced completely into the lumen of the vein.
9. Once the cannula is totally advanced into the vein, the tourniquet is released and digital pressure is applied beyond the cannula tip and the hub stabilized.
10. Fix and apply safety tape, tape is not required for intravenous injection.

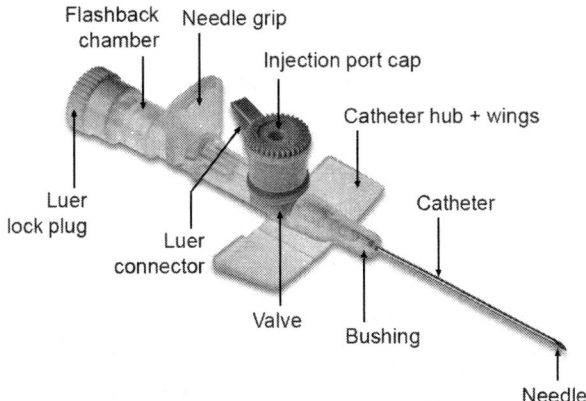

Fig. 12.18: Showing parts of IV cannula

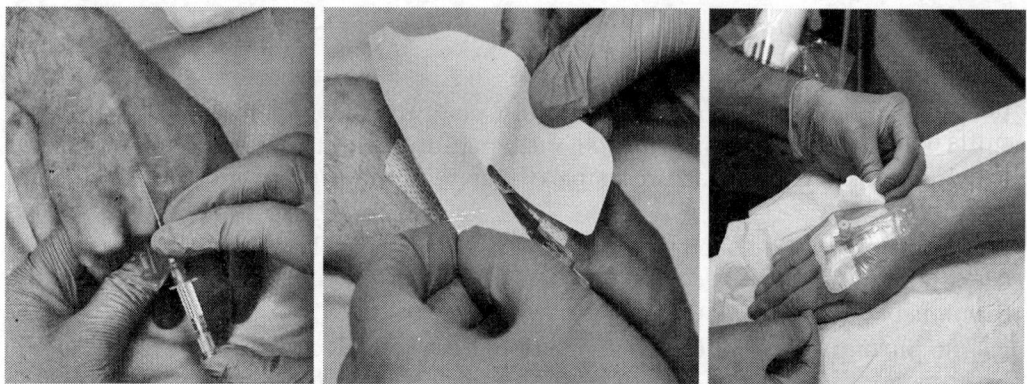

Fig. 12.19: Showing insertion technique of intravenous cannula

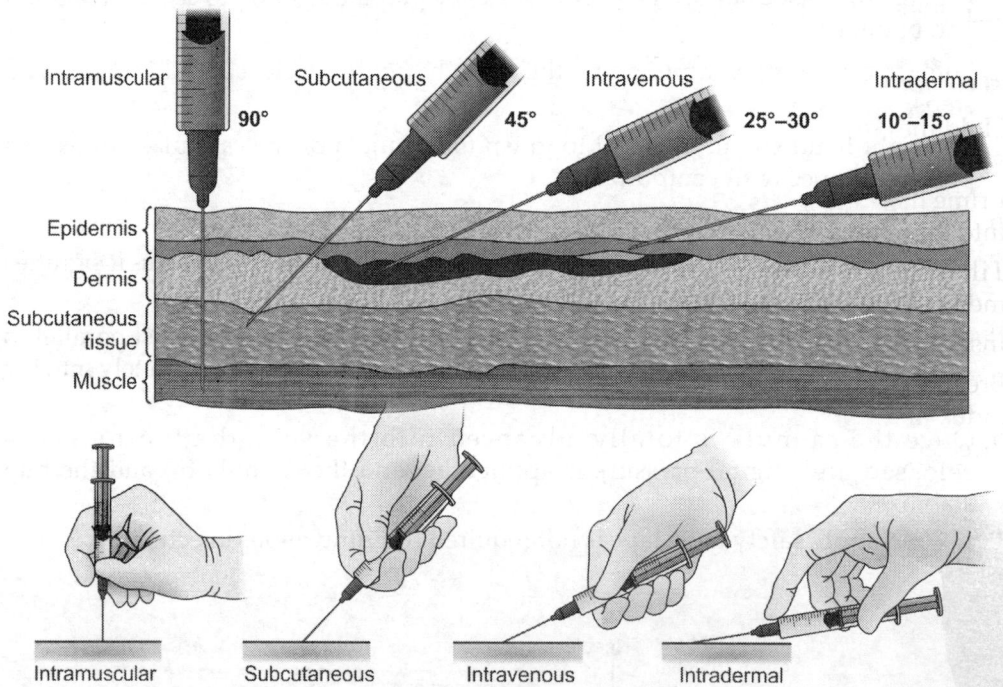

Fig. 12.20: Showing techniques of administration of drug by various parenteral route

How to Use Inhaler

1. Wash your hands thoroughly with soap and warm water.
2. Remove the cap and hold the inhaler upright. Shake the inhaler.
3. Breathe out slowly through your mouth.
4. Hold your inhaler as shown in the picture or as recommended by doctor.
5. While you are breathing in, press down on inhaler one time to release medication.

6. Continue to breathe in slowly and as deeply as you can.

7. Hold your breath for 10 seconds, if you can, to allow the medication to reach deeply into your lungs. Repeat steps 3 to 8 until you have inhaled the number of puffs that your doctor prescribed.

8. Rinse your mouth thoroughly with water. Spit out the water. Do not swallow.

Using a Nasal Spray

1. Close the nostril that is not receiving the medication. Do this by gently pressing on that side of your nose.

2. Gently insert the bottle tip into the other nostril.

3. Breathe in deeply through that nostril as you squeeze the bottle. Remove the bottle and sniff once or twice.

4. Repeat if directed. Wait at least 10 seconds between sprays. If directed, repeat steps 1–4 for the other nostril.

Using a Pump Nasal Spray

1. Hold the bottle with your index and middle fingers on each side of the bottle and your thumb on the bottom of the bottle.

2. Prime the bottle. This is typically done by spraying the product one or more times into the air or into a tissue.

3. Tilt your head slightly forward. Close the nostril that is not receiving the medication. Do this by gently pressing on that side of your nose.

4. Insert the tip of the bottle into the other nostril.

5. Breathe in deeply through that nostril as you press down on the pump with your index and middle fingers. Remove the bottle and sniff once or twice. Repeat if directed. Wait at least 10 seconds between sprays.

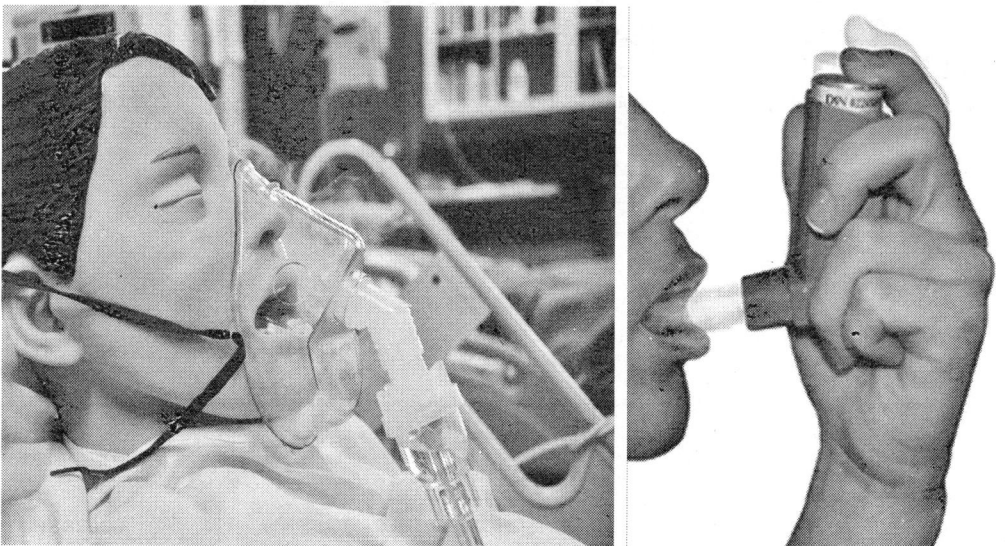

Fig. 12.21: Showing inhalational technique

6. If directed, repeat steps 3–6 for the other nostril.

7. Wait a few minutes to blow your nose after using the nasal spray.

How to Use the Transdermal Patches

1. Wash your hands with soap and water.

2. Select an area of skin to apply the patch. Be sure to follow any specific instructions provided by your doctor or the product instructions as to site selection or rotation.

3. Take the patch out of the packaging. Remove the protective liner on the patch as directed by the patch instructions. Be careful not to touch the sticky side of the patch.

   Note: If the patch's protective liner contains two parts, first peel off one part of the liner. Apply the exposed sticky part of the patch to the skin and press down. Next, peel back the second part of the liner and press the entire patch down.

4. Place the patch, sticky side down, onto the clean, dry and unbroken area of skin. Using the palm of your hand, press down on the patch to make sure the patch is firmly attached to your skin.

5. Use your fingers to press along the edges of the patch. The patch should be smooth, with no bumps or folds.

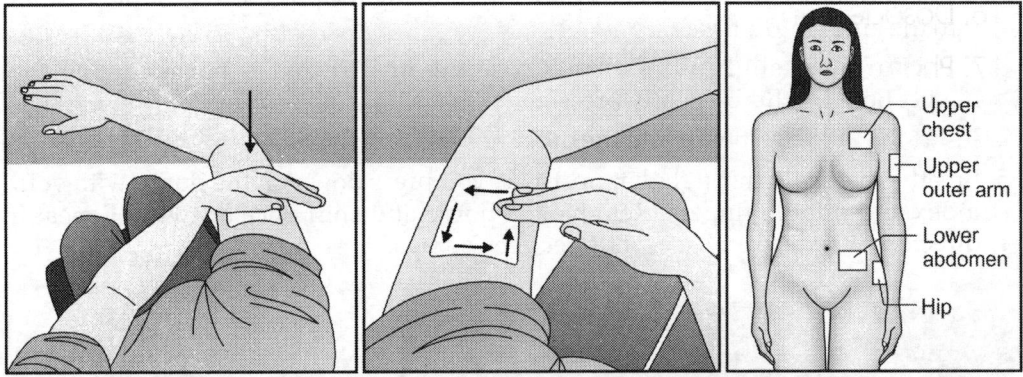

Fig. 12.22: Showing techniques to use transdermal patch

Clinical Pharmacy

13. Introduction to Pharmacy

14. Standard Abbreviations

15. Route of Drug Administration

16. Dosage Forms

17. Pharmacy Preparations

Introduction to Pharmacy

The art and science of preparing and dispensing medicine so as to make them suitable for administration to a patient. Importance of pharmacy is to know the art of dispensing medicine and advances in pharmaceutical industry. The art of identifying selecting, preserving, and combining, analyzing, standardizing, preparing, compounding and dispensing medicine to make them suitable for easy, effective and palatable administration is known as pharmacy.

Pharmacy can be divided into several branches some of which includes pharama-cognosy, analytical pharmacy, manufacturing pharmacy, pharmaceutics and dispensing pharmacy. One of the prerequisites for the practice of pharmacy is the knowledge of metrology.

The present medical practitioners concern with the knowledge of pharmacy is now limited to the knowledge about the nomenclature of the dosage forms. The purity and standard of their contents and the merits and demerits of formulations so as to choose a proper dosage form for the patient.

Definition and Terminologies in Pharmacy

1. **Posology:** Science which deals with doses of drugs.
2. **Materia medica:** Deals with sources, description and preparations of drugs.
3. **Metrology:** Science of weight and measures.
4. **Drug:** WHO defines drug as any substance or product that is used or is intended to be used to modify or explore physiological systems or pathological states for benefit of the recipient.
5. **Dose:** It is the amount of drug given at a time and which can be repeated at defined intervals to produce desired therapeutic effects.
6. **Essential medicines:** According to WHO, essential medicine are those that satisfy the healthcare needs of majority of the population, e.g. iron and folic acid preparations for anaemia in pregnancy.
7. **Orphan drug:** Drugs that are used for diagnosis, treatment or prevention of rare diseases, e.g. Digoxin antibody for digoxin toxicity, Fomepizole for methyl alcohol poisoning.
8. **Over the counter drugs:** OTC or nonprescription drug are the drug that can be sold to a patient without the need for a doctor's prescription, e.g. Paracetamol, Antacids.

9. **Prescription drugs:** These are the drugs that can be obtained only upon producing a prescription by a registered medical practitioner, e.g. antibiotics, atipsychotics.

10. **Adjuvant:** Other active drugs to assist the action of the principal active drug (basis).

11. **Correctives:** Substance added to make the formulation acceptable or to correct some undesirable action of the basis, e.g. sweetening agents, flavouring agents, colouring agents.

12. **Vehicle/excipient/base:** It is the medium in which the active ingredients are distributed.

13. **Draught:** It is a single effective dose of a mixture.

14. **Syrup (IP 1985):** It is a saturated solution of sugar (66% sucrose in water), e.g. simple syrup, codeine phosphate syrup, cyproheptadine syrup.

15. **Elixir (BP 1966):** It is a sweetened and flavored alcoholic solution containing not more than 20% alcohol, e.g. Elixir promethazine.

16. **Oxymel:** It is honey with dilute acetic acid.

17. **Tincture (BP 1980):** It is an alcoholic solution of a nonvolatile substance (70–90% alcohol), e.g. compound tincture of cardamom, tincture benzoin, tincture ipecacuanha, tincture catechu.

18. **Spirit (BP 1980):** It is an alcoholic or hydro alcoholic solution of volatile substances, e.g. aromatic spirit of ammonia, spirit of chloroform.

19. **Aromatic water:** A very weak simple solution of a volatile substance in distilled water, e.g. camphor water, chloroform water.

20. **Infusion:** Prepared by immersing vegetable substances in hot or cold water. They are not subjected to boiling.

21. **Decoction:** Prepared by boiling vegetable substance in water.

22. **Dry extract:** Made by evaporating the solvent of the fluid extract.

23. **Fluid extract:** Liquid alcoholic preparations of definite strength made by percolation.

24. **Bioavailability:** It is the extent and rate of absorption of the drug from a dosage form or as the fraction of the drugs that reaches the site of action.

25. **Bioequivalence:** It is a pharmaceutical equivalent which is not significantly different with respect to rate and extent of absorption in different biological fluids when administred at the same molar dose of the therapeutic ingredients, under similar experimental condition in either single or multiple doses.

26. **Pharmaceutical/chemical equivalence:** These are drug product, which contain equal amount of the same active ingredient but may contain different inactive ingredients.

27. **Therapeutic equivalence:** These are drug products that contain the same therapeutically active drug and give identical effects *in vivo*.

Sources of Information about Drugs

1. **Pharmacopoeia:** This is an official body containing a selected list of medicinal substance and commonly uses with description of their pharmacological category, physiochemical properties, identification and assay technique, storage condition, etc.

These are officially published by an authority of recognized body constituted by law in a particular nation to ensure uniformity of composition and strength of medicines used in treatment of various diseases. These publications are revised periodically, e.g. British Pharmacopoeia (BP), Indian Pharmacopoeia (IP), International Pharmacopoeia (PI), United States Pharmacopoeia (USP), Swiss Pharmacopoeia (SP).

2. **Extra-pharmacopoeia martindale:** It includes both official and nonofficial drugs with their pharmaceutical information, important action, adverse effects, uses with doses and proprietary preparation. Also contains abstracts and technical literature. It gives comprehensive information about the drugs and hence is used widely.

3. **Remington pharmaceutical sciences:** It is a treatise on the theory and practice of pharmacy with essential information about pharmaceutical and medicinal agents, it is a textbook and reference work for pharmacist, physicians and medical scientists.

4. **Other publication:** Indian national formulary, British pharmaceutical codex (BPC), United states dispensary (USD).

5. **Books giving information:** Current Index of Medical Specialities (CIMS), Monthly Index of Medical Specialities (MIMS), Indian Pharmaceutical Guide (IPG), Drug Today.

Metrology

Metrology is defined as science of weights and measures. The word Metrology is derived from greek word 'Metrn' meaning measure. Solids are weighted and liquids are measured. There are two systems of weights and measures (1) The Imperical system (2) The Metric system. Imperical system is an old system based on arbitrary and unrelated units, e.g. grains, drachms, ounces and gallons, whereas the metric system or decimal system is based on related and rationally derived units, e.g. milligrams, grams, centimeters, meters, milliliters, litres, etc. because of its easier calculations, greater accuracy and flexibility and use in other sciences, now-a-days this is the most widely used system by official agencies.

In 1948, a committee on weights and measures legislation was appointed by the president of the Board of Trade to review the existing weights and measures legislation and to make recommendations. In 1951, the committee published a report in which it was recommended that the imperial system should be abolished and the metric system should be adopted in its place. Therefore, steps were taken to abolish the use of imperial system for all dealings in drugs and medicines and its use was declared illegal in pharmacy profession. Accordingly the first change over to the metric system appeared in the British Pharmacopoeia (BP) and British Pharmaceutical Codex published in 1963. The doses of tablet, capsule and injection were given only in metric quantities, due to the above mentioned reasons. Further the patient usually measures the drugs prescribed so carefully by the physician (in mg or ml) with convenient domestic measures like teaspoons, the size of which varies considerably. This system of measurement is called the domestic system.

Weight: It is a measure of the gravitational force acting on a body and is directly proportional to its mass. In metric system, standard unit of measures of mass (weight) is kilogram and all other measures of mass are derived from kilogram.

1 kilogram (kg) = 1000 grams (gm)
1 hectogram (hg) = 100 gm
1 decagram (dag) = 10 gm
1 gram (gm) = 1000 milligram (mg)
1 decigram (dg) = 100 mg
1 centigram (cg) = 10 mg
1 milligram (mg) = 1000 microgram (μg, mcg)
1 microgram (μg, mcg) = 1000 nanogram (ng)
1 nanogram (ng) = 1000 picogram (pg)

Measure: It is the measurement of volume of any substance. The standard unit for measures of capacity (volume) is litre and all other measures of capacity are derived from litre.

1 litre = 1000 millilitre (ml)
1 millilitre = 1000 microlitres (μl)

Domestic Measures: Some household measures are frequently used to measure the doses from the container. Generally, these measures are printed on labels as a direction to be patients. This is convenient to the patients as these measures are commonly available.

1 drop = 0.06 ml
1 teaspoonful = 4 ml
1 desert spoonful = 8 ml
1 tablespoonful = 15 ml
2 tablespoonful = 30 ml
1 wine glassful = 60 ml
1 teacupful = 120 ml
1 tumblerful = 240 ml

Basic Data for Percentage Calculation (Metric System)

Weight/weight 1 gm of solution in 100 gm of solution is 1% w/w. The quantities of electrolytes administered to patients are usually expressed in terms of milliequivalent (mEq) because in this case the electrical activity of ions is important and not the weight in mg or gram.

The formula for calculating milliequivalents/litre is as follows:

$$mEq/L = \frac{mg\% \times 10 \times valancy}{atomic\ wt.}$$

Basic data for calculating percentage: Problem involving calculations of percentage are continuously encountered by the pharmacist. The percentage concentrations of solutions are expressed as follows:

1. **Weight/Weight:** 1 gm of solute in 100 gm of solvent or carrier = 1% W/W.
   e.g. O R S powder, electral powder, ENO powder.
2. **Weight/Volume:** 1 gm of solute in 100 ml solvent = 1% W/V.
   e.g. Vitamin preparation, cough syrups.
3. **Volume/Volume:** 1 part of volume in 100 parts of volume.
   e.g. Alcohol and water.

The percentage calculation

1% solution = 1 : 100
0.1% solution = 1 : 1000
1 in million = 1 : 1,00,000

International units: This is used for expressing quantities of vitamins, e.g. vit A, E and D, antibiotics, e.g. benzyl penicillin sodium, hormones, e.g. insulin, thrombolytics (fibrinolytic), e.g. Streptokinase.

Compounding and dispensing of drugs: This process is carried out in the following order:

1. Reading the prescription.
2. Checking it for patient's safety.
3. Checking for any incompatibilities.
4. Compounding the preparation.
5. Packing the preparation.
6. Labeling it appropriately.
7. Dispensing the preparation.

Apparatus Required

1. Dispensing balance or prescription balance
2. Glass measures
3. Pestle and mortar
4. Ointment slab
5. Spatula
6. Stirrer
7. Dispensing bottles (coloured and colourless)
8. Glue and labelling paper.

Dispensing balance: It is also known as prescription balance.

1. Before use ensures that the pans are clean and pointer is on the zero mark of the scale of dispensing balance.
2. Powdered chemicals and liquids should be weighed on a weighed glass or in a weighing tube, but not directly on the pan.
3. See that the beam is not in motion while putting or removing an object or a weight from pan.
4. Always use forceps for lifting a weight.
5. Put weights on right hand pan and the drugs on the left hand pan.
6. It is reasonably accurate and can weight with (±5% ERROR).
7. It cannot measure quantities less than 50 mg for which a chemical balance may be used.

Glass Measures

1. Conical or cylindrical glass measures are used for measuring the solvents and solutes.

2. These are available in capacities from 5 ml to 1000 ml.
3. Lesser quantities are measured with help of graduate pipettes.

Pestle and Motar

1. It is used for grinding and mixing the ingredients.
2. Made up of porcelain and glass.
3. Used for crushing solid ingredients to powdered form.

Spatula

1. These are made of wood bone or steel.
2. They are used to pour out drugs from container.
3. They are also used for mixing powdered drugs.
4. These are also helpful in spreading plasters.

Supply

1. Mixture in flat white dispensing bottle.
2. Liniment and lotions in corrugated surface blue/brown bottle.
3. Powder in paper wrapper, in envelops.
4. Ointment in pots.
5. Pills in pill box.

Chapter 14

Standard Abbreviations

Meaning of some Latin abbreviation and words: Latin is no more used as a language for prescriptions but the classical influence persists in a number of abbreviations. The use of these abbreviations is not recommended but they are widely used. A few of these are as follows:

Sr. No.	Abbreviation	Latin	Meaning
1	Aa	Ana	Of each
2	Ad	Ad	To, upto
3	ad lib	Ad libitum	To the desired amount
4	a.c.	Ante cibos	Before meals
5	Aq	aqua	Water
6	Aqdest	Aqua destillata	Distilled water
7	b.i.d or b.d.	Bis in die	Twice a day
8	c.	Cum	With
9	co.	compositus	Compound
10	div.	divide	Divide
11	dil.	dilutus	Dilute
12	elix.	elixir	an elixir
13	emp.	emplastrum	A plaster
14	emul.	emulsum	An emulsion
15	et.	Et	And
16	ft.	Fiat	Let it be made
17	gtt.	gutta, guttae	A drop, drops
18	h.s.	hora somni	At bed time
19	Mist.	Mistura	A mixture
20	o.d.	omni die	Daily (once a day)
21	p.c.	post cibos	After meals
22	pil.	pilula	Pill
23	pulv.	pulvis	Powder
24	q.s.	quantum sufficient	A sufficient quantity
25	q.i.d.	Quarter in die	Four times a day
26	q.h.	Quaque hora	Every hour
27	ss.	Semis	Half
28	sig.	Signa	Let it be marked
29	S.O.S	Si opus sit	If necessary
30	Stat.	Statim	Immediately
31	t.i.d(td)	Ter to die	Three times a day
32	M.ft. Mist	Miscefiatmistura	Mixed to make a mixture
33	Tal	talis	Of such

Route of Drug Administration

Routes of drug administration: Most of the drugs can be administered by different routes. Drug- and patient-related factors determine the selection of routes for drug administration. The factors are:

1. Characteristics of the drug.
2. Emergency/routine use.
3. Site of action of the drug-local or systemic.
4. Condition of the patient (unconscious, vomiting, diarrhea).
5. Age of the patient.
6. Effect of gastric pH, digestive enzymes and first-pass metabolism.
7. Patient's/doctor's choice.

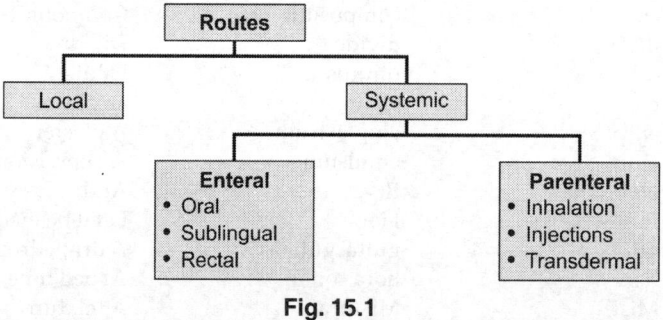

Fig. 15.1

Local Routes

Site: Administration of a drug at the site where the desired action is required.

Examples with dosage form: Antifungal pessaries in vaginal candidiasis, 10% lignocaine hydrochloride for topical anaesthesia.

Advantages

Safe and convenient

Disadvantages

Difficulty in ascertaining the amount of drug absorbed.

Topical: Drug is applied to the skin or mucous membrane at various sites for local action.

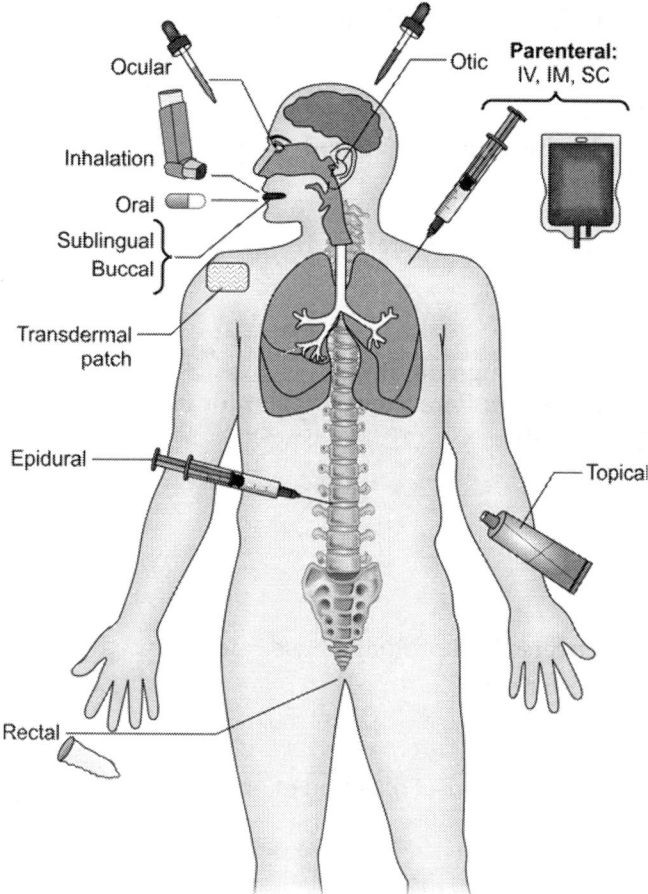

Fig. 15.2

1. **Oral cavity:** For example, Acyclovir cream for herpes labialis, 5% Lignocaine Hydrochloride ointment and jelly for topical anaesthesia, 10% Lignocaine Hydrochloride spray for topical anaesthesia.
2. **GI tract:** As tablet that is not absorbed, e.g. Neomycin for sterilization of gut before surgery.
3. **Rectum and anal canal:**
   a. *As an enema (administration of drug into the rectum in liquid form):*
      Evacuant enema (for evacuation of bowel): For example, soap water enema: soap acts as a lubricant and water stimulates the rectum.
      Retention enema: For example, Methylprednisolone in ulcerative colitis.
   b. As a suppository (administration of the drug in a solid form into the rectum), e.g. Bisacodyl for evacuation of bowels.
4. **Eye, ear and nose:** For example Gentamicin eye/ear drops for infection, allergic conditions, etc.
5. **Bronchi:** For example Salbutamol, Ipratropium bromide inhalation for bronchial asthma and chronic obstructive pulmonary disease.

6. **Skin:** For example, Clotrimazole ointment, cream, lotion (antifungal) for cutaneous candidiasis.

Systemic Routes

Drugs administered by this route enter blood and produce systemic effects.

Enteral Routes

It includes oral, sublingual and rectal routes. (Enteron is a greek word, meaning intestine)

Oral Route

Site: Swallowing a drug through mouth.
Examples with dosage form: Paracetamol tablet for fever, Omeprazole capsule for peptic ulcer are given orally.

Advantages

1. Safer.
2. Cheaper.
3. Painless.
4. Convenient for repeated and prolonged use.
5. Can be self-administered.

Disadvantages

Not suitable for emergency as onset of action of orally administered drugs is slow.

It is not suitable for/in:

1. Unpalatable and highly irritant drugs.
2. Unabsorbable drugs (e.g. aminoglycosides).
3. Drugs that are destroyed by digestive juices (e.g. insulin).
4. Drugs with extensive first-pass metabolism (e.g. lignocaine).
5. Unconscious patients.
6. Uncooperative and unreliable patients.
7. Patients with severe vomiting and diarrhoea.

Sublingual/Buccal Route

Site: The preparation is placed under the tongue or crushed in mouth and spread over the buccal mucosa.

Examples with dosage form: Nitroglycerin tablets for acute anginal attack and Nifedipine capsule for hypertension.

Advantages

1. Quick onset of action.
2. Action can be terminated by spitting out the tablet.
3. Bypasses first-pass metabolism.
4. Self-administration is possible.

Disadvantages

1. **It is not suitable for:** Irritant and lipid-insoluble drugs and drug with higher molecular weight (e.g. insulin).
2. Drugs with bad smell and taste.

Rectal Route

Site: Through rectum.

Examples with dosage form: Glycerine suppositories, enema and ointments for constipation (local effects), Indomethacin suppositories for rheumatoid arthritis (systemic effects).

Advantages

1. Useful in patient having nausea and vomiting.
2. Little or no first pass effect (external haemorrhoidal vein).
3. **It is suitable for:** Irritant drugs.

Disadvantages

1. Inconvenient and embarrassing to the patient.
2. Absorption is slow and erratic.
3. Irritation or inflammation of rectal mucosa can occur

Parenteral Routes

Routes of administration other than enteral route are called parenteral routes. (Par is a greek word meaning aside from). It includes injection, inhalation and transdermal routes.

Advantages

1. Onset of action of drugs is faster; hence it is suitable for emergency.
2. Bioavailability is faster and more predictable.
3. **Useful in:** Unconscious, uncooperative and unreliable patients, patients with vomiting and diarrhoea.
4. **It is suitable for:** Irritant drugs, drugs with high first-pass metabolism, drugs not absorbed orally, drugs destroyed by digestive juices.
5. There are no chances of interference by food or digestive enzymes.
6. Liver enzymes are by-passed.

Disadvantages

1. Require aseptic conditions.
2. Preparation should be sterile and expensive.
3. Requires invasive techniques that are painful.
4. Cannot be usually self-administered.
5. Can cause local tissue injury to nerves, vessels, etc.

Parenteral dosage forms are commonly dispensed in:

1. Ampoules are thin walled glass/plastic containers,which are sealed by fusion of the glass/plastic after filling. The contents should be withdrawn after breaking the seal, on occasion only, e.g. Adrenaline ampoule.
2. **Vials and bottles:** These are thick walled container which are sealed after by a stopper made of material other than glass like plastic, cork or elastomers. The contents may be removed on one or more occasions, e.g. Cefotaxime (single dose vial), Triple antigen (10 dose vial)
3. **Pouches:** Large quantities of intravenous infusion fluids available in collapsible plastic pouches, e.g. normal saline infusion fluid.

Injections

1. Intradermal (Intracutaneous) Route

Site: Injection into the layers of the skin.

Examples with dosage form: Bacillus Calmette-Guerin (BCG) vaccination, diagnostic test and drug sensitivity tests.

Disadvantages

It is painful and only a small amount of the drug can be administered.

2. Subcutaneous (SC) Route

Site: Injection into the subcutaneous tissues of the thigh, abdomen and arm.

Examples with dosage form: Insulin, adrenalin injection (systemic effect) and local anaesthetics (local effects).

Advantages

1. Self-administration is possible (e.g. insulin).
2. Slow absorption for longer period compared to intravenous or intramuscular route.
3. Depot preparations can also be given (e.g. norplant for contraception).

Disadvantages

1. It is suitable for: small volumes of drugs (maximum 2 ml), only for nonirritant drugs.
2. Drug absorption is slow; hence it is not suitable for emergency (e.g. state of shock as decreased peripheral circulation).

Hypodermoclysis is the SC administration of large volume of saline employed in pediatric practice.

Other forms of subcutaneous route include: Pellet implantation, e.g. testosterone, dermoject, e.g. vaccines and sialistic implants, e.g. harmones and contraceptives.

3. Intramuscular (IM) Route

Site: Injection into one of the large skeletal muscles such as deltoid, triceps, gluteus and rectus femoris.

For infants, rectus femoris is used instead of gluteus because gluteus is not well developed till the child starts walking.

Examples with dosage form: Various antibiotics, antiemetics and depot injection of testosterone, haloperidol.

Advantages

1. Absorption is more predictable and rapid as compared to oral route.
2. Mild irritants, depot injections, soluble substances and suspensions can be given by this route.

Disadvantages

1. Aseptic conditions are needed.
2. Intramuscular injections are painful and may cause abscess.
3. Chances of nerve damage.
4. Large volumes cannot be administered. (maximum of 5 ml)

4. Intravenous (IV) Route

Site: Injection into one of superficial vein.

Examples with dosage form: Administered as:

1. **Bolus:** IV Ranitidine in bleeding peptic ulcer.
2. **Slow intravenous injection:** IV Morphine in myocardial infarction.
3. **Intravenous infusion:** Dopamine infusion in cardiogenic shock; mannitol infusion incerebral oedema; fluids infused intravenously in dehydration.

Advantages

1. Bioavailability is 100%.
2. Quick onset of action; therefore, it is the route of choice in emergency, e.g. intravenous Diazepam to control convulsions in status epilepticus.
3. Large volume of fluid can be administered, e.g. intravenous fluids in patients with severe dehydration.
4. Highly irritant drugs, e.g. anticancer drugs can be given because they get diluted in blood.
5. Hypertonic solution can be infused by intravenous route, e.g. 20% mannitol in cerebral oedema.
6. By IV infusion, a constant plasma level of the drug can be maintained, e.g. dopamine infusion in cardiogenic shock.
7. Rapid dose adjustments are possible.

Disadvantages

1. Once the drug is injected, its action cannot be halted.
2. Local irritation may cause phlebitis.
3. Self-medication is not possible.
4. Strict aseptic conditions are needed.

5. Extravasation of some drugs can cause injury, necrosis and sloughing of tissues.

6. Depot preparations cannot be given by IV route.

5. Intrathecal Route

Site: Injection into subarachnoid space.

Examples with dosage form: Xylocaine injection for providing spinal anaesthesia, Amphotericin B injection for cryptococcal meningitis.

Disadvantages

1. Strict aseptic conditions and great expertise are needed.

2. Painful and risky procedure.

6. Intraarticular Route

Site: Injection into joint space.

Examples with dosage form: Hydrocortisone injection for rheumatoid arthritis.

Advantages

Ensures higher concentration of drug in localized area.

Disadvantages

1. Strict aseptic conditions are needed.

2. Painful procedure.

3. Repeated administration may cause damage to the articular cartilage.

7. Intraarterial Route

Site: Injection into arteries.

Examples with dosage form: Radiopaque contrast media for coronary and cerebral angiography, anticancer drugs to treat malignancy.

Advantages

Greater concentration of drug can be delivered at the desired site of action.

Disadvantages

Strict aseptic conditions and great expertise are needed.

8. Intraperitoneal Route

Site: Injection into peritoneal space.

Examples with dosage form: Peritoneal dialysis in case of poisoning and renal failure.

Advantages

Rapid absorption due to larger surface area

Disadvantages

1. Strict aseptic conditions are needed.

2. Painful and risky due to chances of adhesions and infections in peritoneal cavity.

9. Intramedullary Route

Site: Injection into tibial or sterna bone marrow. Now rarelyin use

Examples with dosage form: Bone marrow transplantation.

Advantages
Rapid onset of action.

Disadvantages
Strict aseptic conditions, painful, risky great expertise are needed.

Inhalation

Site: Inspiration through nose or mouth.

Examples with dosage form: Volatile liquids and gases are given by inhalation for systemic effects, e.g. general anaesthetics, e.g. Metered aerosol preparations of salbutamol for the treatment of bronchial asthma.

Advantages
1. Quick onset of action.
2. Dose required is very less, so systemic toxicity is minimized.
3. Amount of drug administered can be regulated.

Disadvantages
1. Local irritation may cause increased respiratory secretions and bronchospasm.
2. Important route of entry of certain drugs of abuse.
3. Drug particles may induce cough (e.g. cromolyn sodium)

Transdermal Route

Site: Adhesive matrix (patch) containing drug is applied to chest, upper abdomen or mastoid region.

Examples with dosage form: Scopolamine patch for motion sickness, Nitroglycerin patch/ointment for angina, Oestrogen patch for hormone replacement therapy (HRT).

Advantages
1. Duration of action is prolonged.
2. Systemic side effects are reduced.
3. Provide a constant plasma concentration of the drug.

Disadvantages
4. Expensive.
5. Local irritation may cause dermatitis and itching.
6. Patch may fall-off unnoticed.

Dosage Forms

The science of dosage forms and their design is known as *pharmaceutics*. Dosage form is the finished product by means of which drugs are actually administered to the patients for diagnostic, prophylactic or therapeutic purpose.

Dosage form are the devices into which drug substances can be incorporated for the convenient and efficacious treatment of a disease. These devices require pure drug alongwith various nondrug component called excipient or adjuvant. The selection of excipients should be such that it does not alter the properties of the pure drug in a dosage form. The processing techniques, which include various pharmaceutical operations like size reduction, mixing, granulation, compression, etc. may also play an important role in increasing or decreasing the efficacy and stability of dosage forms. Dosage forms can be designed for administration of a drug by all possible routes to achieve maximum therapeutics response.

The route of administration of a drug is also important in optimizing drug therapy and from the patients point of view it becomes necessary to administer drugs in a way that is least uncomfortable today, a number of dosage forms are available to suit every conceivable route and application.

The need for dosage forms:

1. Accurate dose

2. Protection, e.g. coated tablets, sealed ampoules

3. Protection from gastric juice

4. Masking taste and odour

5. Placement of drugs within body tissues

6. Sustained release medication

7. Controlled release medication

8. Optimal drug action

9. Insertion of drugs into body cavities (rectal, vaginal)

10. Use of desired vehicle for insoluble drugs.

Table 16.1: Classification of dosage form as per route of administration

Route of administration	Site	Dosage form
Oral	Mouth	Solution, syrup, elixirs, suspension, emulsion, creams, gels, powders, granules, capsules, tablets, pills, cachets
Sublingual	Below the tongue	Sublingual tablet
Parenteral	Below some or other layer of skin-subcutaneous. intravenous, intra-arterial	Solution, suspension, emulsion, powder, implants, inhalations, sprays, gases
Rectal	Rectum	Suppositories, ointments, creams, solutions, suspensions, emulsion, enema, tablet
Topical	Skin surface	Ointments, cream, pastes, lotion, liniments, gels, solution, topical aerosols, poultices, collodions
Transdermal	Skin surface	Transdermal patches
Vaginal	Vagina	Passaries, ointments, cream, gel, jellies, solution, douches, emulsion foams, tablet
Nasal	Nose	Solution, inhalation
Ophthalmic	Eye	Solution, suspension ointment, cream, inserts
Otic/aural	Ear	Solution, suspension, powders

Classification as per their Physical State

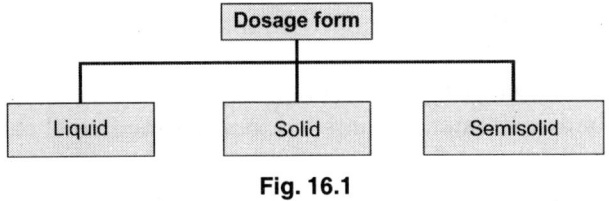

Fig. 16.1

Liquid Dosage Form

Advantages

1. Ease of administration, homogenous.
2. Quick onset of action as compared to solid dosage form.
3. Better bioavaibility as compared to solid dosage form.

Disadvantages

1. Poses stability problem as water is a good medium for hydrolysis reaction, microbial growth. So addition of preservatives is a must for aqueous preparation.
2. Some individuals are sensitive to preservative, may precipitate side effects.
3. Bulky to carry.

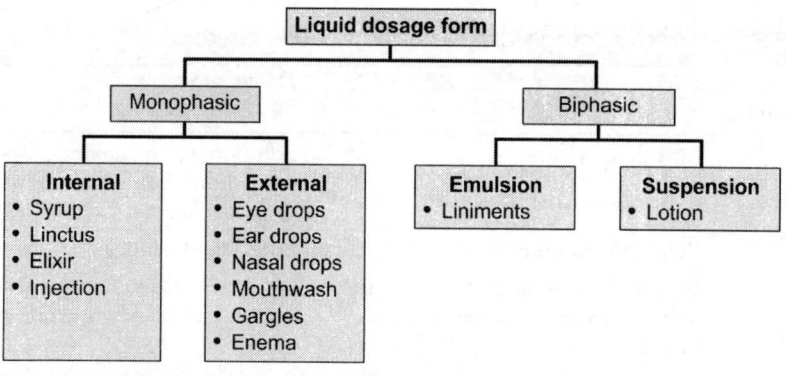

Fig. 16.2

Liquid Dosage form: Monophasic

For Internal Use

1. **Simple mixture:** Liquid preparation containg one or more medicinal substances in dissolved state. These may be solution, suspension or emulsion.
2. **Syrup:** It is a saturated solution of sugar (66% sucrose in water) with or without added flavouring agents and medicinal substances, e.g. simple syrup, Paracetamol syrup, Codeine phosphate syrup, Cyproheptadine syrup
3. **Elixir:** It is a sweetened and flavoured alcoholic solution containg not more than 20% alcohol, e.g. orange elixir, promethazine elixir, phenobarbitone elixir
4. **Draughts:** It is a single effective dose of a mixture.
5. **Linctuses:** Viscous liquid containing high concentration of sucrose usually prescribed for the relief of cough, e.g. Honitus
6. **Drops:** Clear, sweetened and flavored liquids usually formulated for pediatric and dispensed in a suitable bottle containing calibrated dropper.
7. **Tinctures:** Alcoholic or hydroalcoholic solution prepared from vegetable materials or from chemical substances.
8. **Spirit:** It is an alcoholic or hydroalcoholic solution of volatile substances. Spirits are taken internally or sometimes inhaled for their medicinal value, e.g. aromatic spirit of ammonia, spirit of chloroform
9. **Aqua/aromatic water:** Clear, saturated aqueous solution of volatile oils or other aromatic or volatile substances.
10. **Oxymel:** It is honey with dilute acetic acid.
11. **Decoction:** It is prepared by boiling a vegetable substance in water.

For External Use

1. **Liniments:** Alcoholic or oily clear solution intended for application to the skin with friction or massage and should not be applied to broken skin, e.g. Amrutanjan, Iodex
2. **Lotion:** Clear solution may be either aqueous or oily suspension or emulsion for external application without friction, either dabbed on the skin or applied on a suitable dressing and covered with a waterproof dressing to reduce evaporation, e.g. Lactocalamine lotion, sunscreen lotion.

3. **Collodions:** Liquid preparation for external use, usually applied with a brush or rod. The solvent system of collodions is volatile which evaporates.

For Special Use

1. **Ear drops:** Aqueous or oily solution or suspension of one or more medicaments intended to be instilled into the outer ear with a dropper, e.g. Soliwax ear drops.

2. **Eye drops:** Sterile, isotonic, aqueous or oily solution or suspension of one or more medicaments intended to be instilled into the conjunctival sac, e.g. artificial tears

3. **Eye lotions:** Aqueous solution used undiluted for bathing the eye, e.g. Optrex eye lotion.

4. **Nasal drops:** Aqueous solution of drugs intended to be instilled into the nose with a dropper, e.g. Nasoclear, Ortivin nasal drops.

5. **Enemas:** Aqueous solution of drug intended for rectal administration.

6. **Douches:** Medicated solution for rinsing a body cavity. The word douche is most often used for rinsing vaginal cavity.

7. **Gargles:** Aqueous solution employed for local action in the throat. They are dispensed in concentrated form with directions for dilution with lukewarm water before use, e.g. Betadine gargles.

8. **Paints:** Solution in viscous vehicle intended to be applied on the skin or mucosa with some soft device such as brush or cotton

9. **Mouth wash:** Liquid preparation for treating oral infections and bad breath and providing feeling of freshness. They are usually supplied in concentrated form and diluted before use, e.g. Listerine mouth wash.

10. **Irrigation:** Solution of medicament used to treat infections of the bladder, vagina and less often the nose. They are introduced with the help of soft tubes

11. **Sprays:** Aqueous alcoholic or glycerin containg solution of drugs intended to be applied to the mucosa of nose or throat with an atomizer or nebulizer.

12. **Inhalations:** Solution of drugs administered by nasal or oral respiratory route for local or systemic effects, e.g. Asthalin inhaler

13. **Parenterals:** Sterile, pyrogen free preparation containing one or more medications intended to be administer parenterally. The word parenteral is derived from the Greek words para and enteron means outside the intestine and denotes routes of administration other than the oral route.

Liquid Dosage form: Biphasic

For Internal Use

1. **Suspension:** Aqueous or oily coarse dispersions finely, divided insoluble drug suspended in a liquid medium, e.g. Zental suspension, Magmas, Cefixime oral suspension

2. **Emulsion:** These are heterogeneous systems in which one liquid phase is dispersed in the form of minute globules into another immiscible liquids phase. They are also called coarse dispersions of liquids in liquids. Various type of emulsion are O/W and W/O type.

For External Use

1. **Applications:** Suspension or emulsions intended to be applied to the skin.
2. **Liniments:** Emulsion intended for application to the skin with friction or massage they are not applied to the broken skin.
3. **Lotion:** Emulsion or suspension intended to be applied to the skin without friction. They may be applied as such or with the support of suitable dressing material.

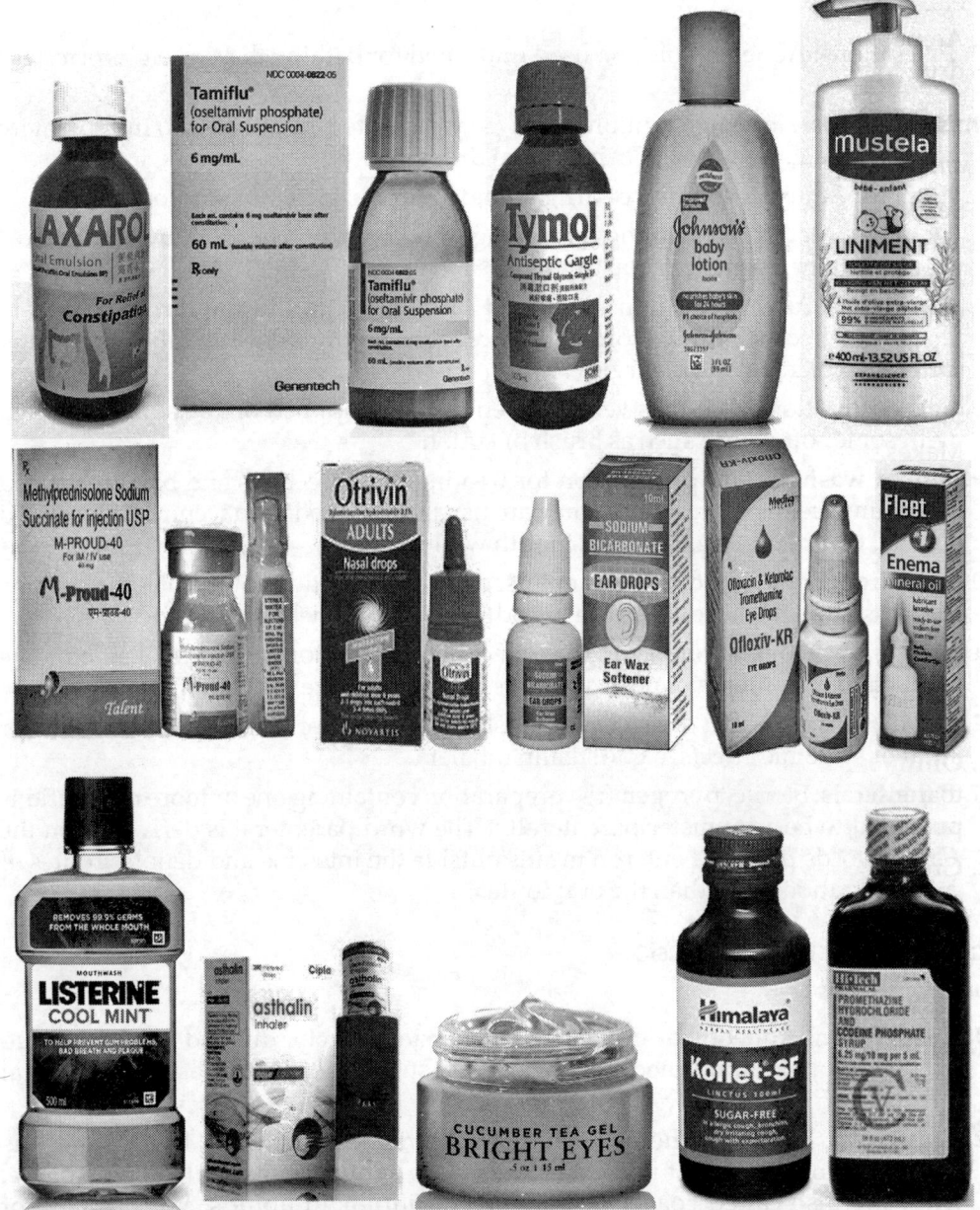

Fig. 16.3: Liquid dosagets form: Marketed product

For Special Use

1. **Enema:** Suspension or emulsions of medicaments intended for rectal administration.
2. **Eye drops:** Suspension of drugs intended to be instilled into conjunctival sac.
3. **Inhalation:** Suspension of volatile oils or substances absorbed on some adsorbing agents. The vapors of volatile substances are inhaled by adding the preparation to hot water or by placing the preparation on an absorbent.
4. **Ear drops:** Suspension or aqueous solution of drugs that are instilled into the ear.
5. **Aerosols:** Suspension of fine solid or liquids particles in a gas are used to apply drug to respiratory tract and skin.

Semisolid Dosage Forms

Advantages

1. Serves as vehicle for carrying medicament for local action as well as systemic action.
2. Remains on applied area for longer time.
3. Quick onset of action for local aliment as compared to oral dosage form.

Disadvantages

1. Stains cloths, skin surface.
2. Makes the surface greasy.

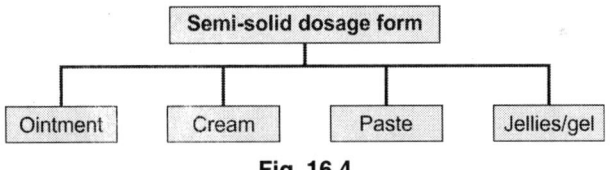

Fig. 16.4

1. **Ointment:** Homogeneous, semisolid preparation intended for external application to the skin or certain mucous membrane for emollient, protective or prophylactic purpose, e.g. Thuja ointment
2. **Cream:** Highly viscous emulsion containing medicinal agents intended for external use.
3. **Paste:** Semisolids preparations containing very high proportion of the solid medicament (20–50%) and intended for topical application, e.g. Colgate tooth paste
4. **Jellies:** Transparent or translucent nongreasy semisolid preparations intended to be used externally.
5. **Plasters:** Solid or semisolid dosage forms adhered to the suitable backing material like cotton, linen, muslin, etc. and intended for external application to a part of the body to provide prolonged contact at the site. They are adhesive at body temperature and the backing material on to which the mass is adhered is cut into different shapes appropriate to cover the affected part.

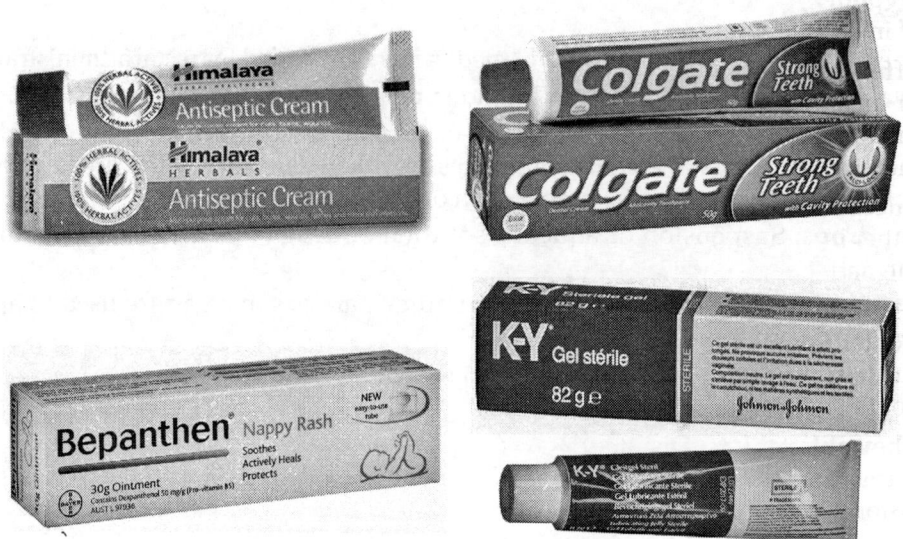

Fig. 16.5: Semisolid dosage form: Marketed products

Solid Dosage Forms

Advantages

1. Most versatile, flexible in strength.
2. Relatively stable chemically, microbiologically.
3. Presents less problem during formulation, packing and storage.
4. Less drug-drug, drug-excipient interaction and interaction with packing.

Disadvantages

1. Onset of action is delayed as compared to liquid dosage form.
2. Paediatric, geriatrics is unable to swallow tablets and capsules.

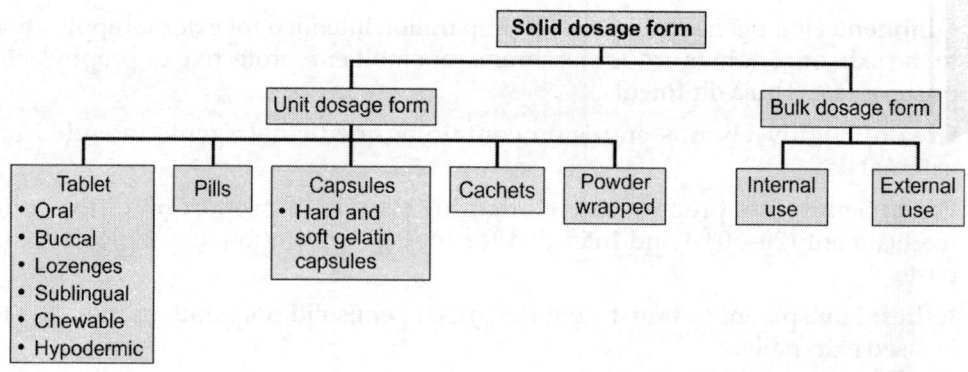

Fig. 16.6: Flowchart showing classification of various solid dosage form

1. Tablet: Solid dosage forms containing one or more medicaments. They can be either moulded or compressed. Moulded tablets are prepared by manual pressure, while compressed tablets are prepared by applying heavy pressure with the help of machinery.

2. **Hypodermal tablets:** Tablets are soluble in water and available for the preparation of injectable solutions.

3. **Effervescent tablets:** Tablets containing acidic substances and either carbonates or bicarbonates which react rapidly in the presence of water to release carbon dioxoide. It is use effervescence as a property to mask the unpleasant taste of medicaments, e.g. Effervescent antacid tablets

4. **Buccal and sublingual tablets:** Small oval dosage forms intended to be inserted either in the gum and the cheek (buccal) or beneath the tongue (sublingual),where the active ingredient is absorbed directly without being required to pass into gastrointestinal tract, e.g. Glyceryl trinitrite, steroidal tablets

5. **Coated tablets:** Tablets covered with one or more layers of mixture of various substances such as resins, gums, inactive and insoluble fillers sugar, plasticisers, polyhydric alcohols, waxes. The coating may also contains medicaments.

6. **Chewable tablets:** Disintegrate smoothly at a satisfactory rate, on chewing. This is due to diluents like mannitol, lactose or inositol, such tablets have a pleasant taste feels no unpleasant aftertaste, e.g. vitamin C and calcium

7. **Lozenges:** Flavoured tablets, which intended to dissolved in the oral slowly. It is intended for treatment of local irritation or infections of the throat or sometimes mouth, but may contain active ingredients intended for systemic absorption after swallowing, e.g. Strepsils, Vicks

8. **Capsule:** Capsule are small, hard or soft soluble, gelation containers intended to be filled with drugs and swallowed, e.g. vitamin E

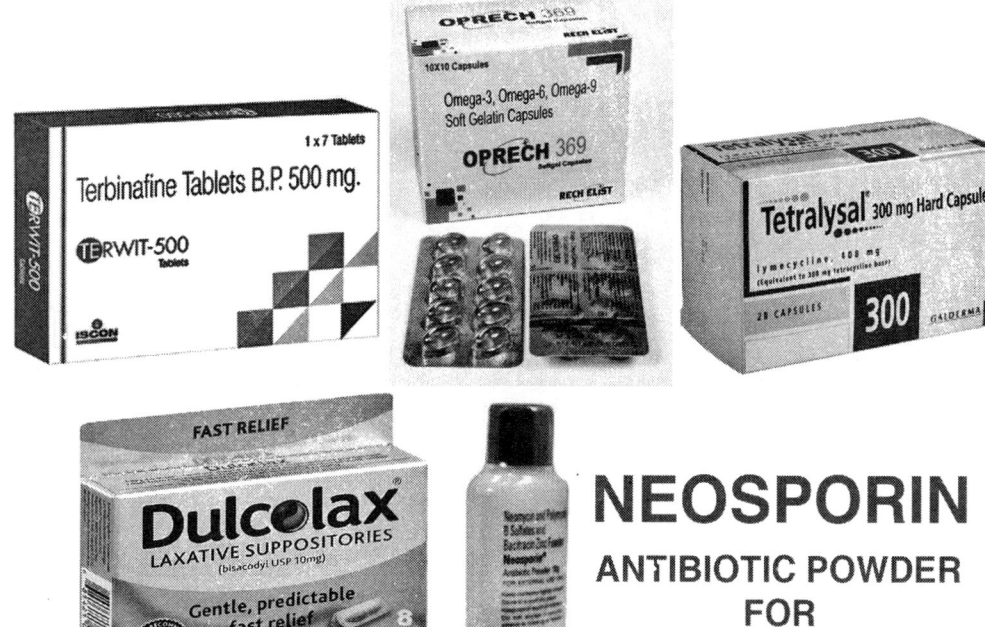

Fig. 16.7: Solid dosage form: Marketed products

9. **Pill:** Oral dosage forms which consist of spherical masses prepared from one or more medicaments incorporated with inert excipients. Pills are now rarely used.

10. **Cachets:** Consist of a dry powder enclosed in a shell. The shell is prepared from a mixture of rice flour and water by moulding into suitable shape and then dried. eg. sodium aminosalicylate catchets, isoniazid cachets

11. **Powder enclosed in capsules:** Powder that are nauseous or bitter in taste are enclosed in capsule, before administration the medicaments suitably powdered with or without dilution is weighted and filled in the body of capsule and cap is pressed on.

12. **Tablet triturates or moulded or compressed powder:** Powder are compressed or moulded in tablet form with the help of lactose or other dilutentslike starch mannitol, dextrose and 60% alcohol they can be swallowed whole or reduced to powder by crushing tablet triturates are useful when powder is required extemporaneously.

13. **Powder:** Powders are finely powdered drugs intended for external use or internal administration, e.g. external use: dusting powders medicated powders Neosporin powder and internal application Oral rehydration salts.

14. **Suppositories:** Solid, uniformly medicated masses intended for introduction into the body cavities, usually having a local action but occasionally a systemic one. It is important that these preparations should retain their moulded shape until body temperature is reached when they should melt or soften and release the medicament Insitu, e.g. glycerine, tannic acid, Belladonna

Pharmacy Preparations

MIXTURES

A mixture is a liquid medicament containing dissolved, suspended or emulsified substances in a suitable vehicle and is meant for internal use. A single, effective dose of a mixture is called a draught, e.g. Piperazine citrate.

Advantages of Mixtures

1. They are more quickly effective than pills or tablets which require disintegration before absorption.
2. Certain substances can be given only as mixture, e.g. Castor oil or Liquid paraffin
3. Certain substances are more effective if given in liquid form, e.g. Bismuth salt or Antacids given in the form of a suspension for peptic ulcer disease.
4. Certain substances are irritant if taken in the dry state (powder or tablet) and may cause pain and therefore are given as mixture, e.g. Potassium iodide and Potassium bromide.
5. They are often more palatable.
6. They are easy to administer.

Requirements of a Good Mixture

1. Ingredient should be uniform and evenly distributed.
2. Activity of one drug should not be administered by combination with another.
3. Soluble substances should not be rendered insoluble.
4. Mixture should be pleasing to the eye and palatable. For this, certain correctives (sweetening, colouring and flavouring agents) may be added.

Type of mixtures

1. Solutions
2. Suspensions
3. Emulsions

Solutions: It is a perfectly homogenous liquid preparation containing one or more substances dissolved in a fluid medium called the solvent.

1. Simple solutions containing soluble solids, e.g. Oral rehydration solution, ferric ammonium

2. Simple solutions containing insoluble solids made soluble with the use of other substances, e.g. mixture of lugols iodine, camphor in alcohol.

Suspension: A suspension is a liquid medicament containing insoluble (diffusible or nondiffusible) substances which are homogeneously distributed throughout the vehicle with or without the help of a suspending agent. Suspension can be given orally, intramuscularly or intravenously or may be used locally.

1. Diffusible substances do not dissolve in water but may be mixed therewith so that upon shaking the solids evenly diffuse throughout the liquid for sufficient time to ensure uniform distribution in each dose, e.g. Mist Alba

2. Nondiffusible substances do not remain evenly distributed in the vehicle long enough to ensure uniformity of the measured dose and hence a suspending agent has to be added. Often dry powder are dispensed so that the suspension can be freshly prepared, e.g. Ampicillin dry powder for suspension.

Suspending agents are pharmacologically inert substances increase the viscosity of the vehicle, which is required to hold a powder in suspension for a given period, e.g. Glycerine, Tragacanth, Acacia, Mucilage of Tragacanth, Mucilage of Acacia

Instruction: It is necessary to write instruction on the label "Shake well before use" (it can be written in bold letters or underlined).

Properties of a Good Suspension

1. After shaking, the medicament stays in suspension long enough for the dose to be accurately measured.
2. The suspension is easily redispersed.
3. Particles in suspension should be small and relatively uniform in size so that the product is not gritty in texture and the suspension can be easily removed from the container.

Emulsion: An emulsion is defined as a system of two immiscible liquids, one of which is finely divided into small globules and dispersed into the other with the help of an emulsifying agent (emulgent). Emulsion can be used for both internal and external administration.

When two immiscible liquids are in contact with one another, there exists at the separating surface or interface, a certain tension or force which retards dispersion of one liquid and are accordingly said to be immiscible. Vigorous shaking may break up one liquid into globules which become temporarily distributed throughout the other liquid, but on standing for some time separation quickly takes place. To avoid this, a third agent called an emulsifying agent is added.

Thus, the three main components of an emulsion are:

1. **Continuous/external phase/dispersion medium:** The liquid that surrounds the globules of liquid in a dispersed phase.
2. **Dispersed/Internal phase/discontinuous phase:** The liquid that is broken into fine globules
3. Emulsifying agent.

Emulsifying agents is a substance, which concentrates as a film at the interface of the two immiscible liquids and thereby lowers the interfacial tension. This helps the dispersion of the dispersed phase into fine globules and prevents it from separating into a different layer. There are many types of emulsifying agents and they can be classified into the following groups. A single emulsifying agent may be used for most dispensing purpose, but it has been proved that two or more agents used together produce finer emulsion and this is the practice in large scale manufacture.

1. Gums-gum acacia, gum tragacanth
2. Soaps-monovalent, divalent alkalies
3. Proteins-casein, gelatin and egg yolk
4. Carbohydrates-maltose
5. Synthetic-carboxy-methyl-cellulose, Tween 80.

Types of Emulsion

1. **Oil in water (O/W)** i.e. oil as dispersed phase and water as continuous phase
2. **Water in oil (W/O)** i.e. water as dispersed phase and oil as continuous phase

Difference between O/W and W/O Type Emulsion

Sr No.	Oil in water (O/W)	Water in oil (W/O)
1	Internal and external administration	Only external application
2	The dispersed phase is oil and the dispersion medium in water.	The dispersed phase is water and the dispersion medium in oil.
3	Milk white appearance	Waxy and translucent appearance
4	Free dilution of water	Free dilution of oil
5	Methylene blue imparts uniform blue colour	Sudan III imparts red colour
6	Conducts electricity	Does not conduct electricity
7	e.g. Turpentine liniment	e.g. Cold creams

Preparation of an Emulsion

While preparing an emulsion, a primary emulsion is prepared by taking the right proportion of oil, water and emulgent. This is then freely diluted with the continuous phase to form the secondary emulsion. A good emulsion is milky white in colour, has a homogenous appearance and if a drop of the emulsion is added to the continuous phase it disperses easily.

Examples of Naturally Occurring Emulsions

1. **Latex:** It is the milky juice of certain plants and consists of an emulsion of rubber in water. The emulgent is the protoid substance.
2. **Egg yolk:** The yellow part of the egg is the oil emulsified by protoid matter egg yolk itself is used as an emulgent under certain condition.
3. **Milk:** The most perfect and naturally occurring emulsion is milk. It contains fat emulsified by the protein known as casein.

Reasons for the Use of Emulsion in Pharmaceutics

1. They facilitate the administration of substances that are immiscible in water.
2. Covering properties of the emulgent mask the bad taste of liquids and make them palatable.
3. In the case of an O/W emulsion, extremely small particles of the dispersed phase (oil) are more effective than if the oil administered in an undivided state.

Steps for Dispensing Mixtures

1. The bottle is calibrated.
2. The ingredients are weighted or measured and a uniform mixture is prepared.
3. The mixture is then transferred to the calibrated bottle.
4. The label, including the dose slip are stuck on the bottle.
5. The bottle is corked and polished to remove finger marks.

Ways to Make Mixture More Acceptable

Mixture are made less offensive and more elegant by altering or modifying their taste and flavor by addition of corrective or corringents.

1. Colour can be modified by using various colouring agents, e.g. tincture cardamom to give a red colour to mixtures.
2. Taste can be masked by adding sweet and/or sour agents or by masking the mixture effervescent. Their disadvantage probably increase in the incidence of dental caries and therefore it is advisable to avoid them as far as possible.

Sweetening agents: These are commonly used in children and include sugar glycerine; the glycyrrhizin (incompatible with acids) and saccharine (1:2000 or 1:100000). These improve alkaline sour or salty taste they do not improve astringent and bitter tastes.

Sour agents: Citric acid and its preparations, e.g. lemon syrup, they improve salty insipid and bitter tastes.

Flavour is taste with smell: Various flavouring agents are available and include:

mild flavor–Lemon, orange, cherry, raspberry, anise and fennel.

strong flavor–Cinnamon, clove, peppermint, cardamom, and ginger.

other flavouring agents–Oil of rose, oil of bitter almonds, lavender, vanillin and balsam.

Liniments

These are liquid preparations containing one or more active ingredients, generally with rubefacient or counter-irritant properties for external application with friction. Unlike lotions, liniments are usually mixtures of dissolved suspended or emulsified ingredients.

Examples

1. **Suspension:** Compound calamine liniment
2. **Emulsion:** Turpentine liniment

White liniment a base for many other liniments contains both dissolved and emulsified components.

Differences between Lotion and Liniment

Sr. No	Lotion	Liniment
1	Applied to skin or mucosa	Applied only to skin
2	Applied without friction	Applied with friction
3	Cooling, smoothing protective properties	Rubefacient counter-irritant, analgesic properties
4	Do not contain camphor	Contains camphor or other irritants

By definition liniments are intended for rubbing into the skin and their oil or soap components increases ease of application and massage. Alcoholic liniments penetrate skin readily than those with an oily base. The oily liniments milder in their action but are more useful when massage is required.

Mechanism of Action of Liniments

Liniments are used for their counterirritant properties which are conferred by the volatile oils used in them by stimulating an area of the skin and they reduce the ascending traffic of pain signals from underlying deeper or visceral structures supplied by the same segments of the spinal cord. This helps to temporarily mask pain from the deeper structures thus liniments are used in various musculoskeletal aches and pains as well as in conditions like sciatica or arthritis. Liniments may contain additional ingredients that confer analgesic, astringent or emollients properties.

Dispensing and Labeling Requisites

Liniments like lotion should be dispensed in fluted bottles clearly labeled "for external use only" liniment should not to be applied to bruised or broken skin.

Lotions

They are liquid preparations containing one or more active ingredients, intended for topical application to skin or mucous membrane, without friction.

Types of lotion

The majority of lotions are for application to unbroken skin. However, some lotion like eye lotions, mouth washes, gargles or vaginal irrigation solution can be applied to the mucosa.

Lotion are usually suspension of solids in an aqueous medium, though some lotions may be solutions or emulsions.

Example

1. **Suspension:** Calamine lotion, hydrocortisone lotion
2. **Solutions:** Povidone iodine solution, Clotrimazole solution
3. **Emulsion:** Benzyl benzoate lotion.

Properties and Uses of Lotions

Lotions, in general, have soothing and protective properties, dermatologists frequently prescribe lotion containing antiseptic, anaesthetic, antihistaminic, antipyretic, astringent, anti-inflammatory or antimicrobial agent and other types of agents like sunscreens for the treatment or prevention of a variety of skin disorders.

Lotions are also widely employed as cleansing preparations for mucosal surfaces as exemplified by eye lotions and mouth washes.

Lotions are stable preparations, unlike semisolid, topical preparations like ointments and creams, can be applied to hairy areas of the body such as the scalp. However, they need to be used in relatively large quantities, especially for cleansing purposes.

Requirements of a Good Lotion

Even though lotions are applied without friction, the insoluble matter they contain must be finely divided and the preparation must be made into a uniform one so that an accurate amount of the dose is applied each time.

1. Particles approaching colloidal dimensions are more smoothing to inflamed areas and more effective when applied to infected surface.
2. Incorporation of glycerine keeps the skin moist for longer periods.
3. Lotion intended to evaporate quickly from the skin surface, the vehicle is usually alcoholic also enhances the cooling effect of a lotion.
4. Excipients in lotions stabilize the preparation, act as preservative or accentuate the cooling, smoothing or protective properties of the active ingredients.
5. Lotions must be prepared and dispensed in an attractive manner, as the cosmetic aspect of lotions is of considerable importance.

Preparation of Lotions

Lotions may be prepared by triturating the ingredients to a smooth paste and then adding the remaining vehicle with continued trituration on a large scale, lotions are prepared by using colloid milk and high-speed mixers which produce better dispersion than is possible by hand.

Dispensing and Labeling Requisites

Lotions are preferably dispensed in oval bottles that are vertically ribbed on the back. This characteristic of the lotion bottle warns the user (in the dark or if he has impaired eyesight) that the contents are not to be taken orally. This is further emphasized by the warning "For external use only" on the label. Patients must also be instructed while dispensing not to apply the lotion to broken skin and to keep inflammable products away from naked flames.

Ointments

Ointments are semisolid greasy preparations for application to the skin or mucous membrane. They are mainly used for their protective and emollient effects. The base used in an ointment is usually anhydrous and contains one or more medicaments.

The consistency and composition of ointments should be such that they may be readily applied to the skin by inunctions and soften but do not melt when applied to the body.

The vehicle of an ointment is known as an ointment base. The choice of the base depends upon the clinical indication for the ointment and the different types of ointment base are:

1. **Hydrocarbon bases:** These have poor penetrability, superficial action and good stability and do not turn rancid. They are used when superficial or simple protective action is desired, e.g. hard paraffin, soft paraffin.
2. **Absorption bases:** Unlike the hydrocarbon type, they are hydrophilic and therefore, can absorb considerable amount of water. They are less occlusive, have better penetrability and are easier to spread, e.g. animal bases like wool fat (anhydrous lanolin), beeswax, hydrous wool fat.
3. **Water soluble bases:** These are water soluble and hence easily removed from the skin. They have excellent penetrability, are non-greasy and spread easily, e.g. macrogols 200, 300, 400

Properties Which Affects Choice of an Ointment Base

1. **Stability:** Hydrocarbon bases are stable while animal bases get rancid after storage.
2. **Penetrability:** Hydrocarbon base are used for superficial action, e.g. in Whitefield's ointment whereas water soluble bases are used when drugs are required to penetrate the skin.
3. **Solvent properties:** For example, for phenol ointment, an animal base is used because phenol is soluble in it. For camphor ointment, olive oil is used.
4. **Irritant effect:** Eye ointment should be free from irritant effects.
5. **Ease of application and removal:** If a the base is sticky, prolonged contact with the skin is ensured. However stickiness makes application difficult and leads to contamination of clothes. Further, if the ointments is applied on a healing wound and gauze covering the wound is removed, the newly formed granulation tissue may get peeled off along with it, retarding healing.

Methods of Preparation of Ointments

Two mixing techniques are frequently used in making ointments.

1. **Trituration:** In this method, finely subdivided insoluble medicaments are evenly distributed by grinding with small amount of the base followed by dilution with gradually increasing amounts of base. Trituration may be performed with a mortar and pestle or with an ointment tile and spatula. It is easier to transfer an ointment to a container from a tile than from a mortar but, if the quantity is rather large or it is necessary to incorporate a liquid, a mortar is more suitable.
2. **Fusion:** In this method, the ingredients are melted together (in descending order of their melting points) and stirred to ensure homogeneity.

Properties of a Good Ointment

A good ointment is homogenous and free of gritty particles, smooth and greasy to feel stable over a period of time and free from microbial contamination.

Dispensing of an Ointment

Ointments are always dispensed with the instructions "for external use only" in butter paper pots, greaseproof boxes or collapsible tubes.

It is difficult to deliver the precise dose of the active ingredient at each application. Several techniques are used to measure the dose of a medicine and include:

1. Weighing the tube or the container before and after application, which is the best method although cumbersome.

2. Measuring the length of the ribbon of ointment squeezed from the tube. This system is used when nitroglycerine ointment is applied for systemic effect.

Powder

A powder is a solid dosage forms, which contains one or more ingredients mixed with each other in a dry and finely divided state. A powder must weigh at least 100 mg. If the quantity is less, it is made upto 100 mg by adding a suitable diluents, e.g. lactose, sodium bicarbonate, magnesium oxide, kaolin. The powders are usually dispensed in sachets or may be wrapped in paper.

Classification of Powders

1. **Simple powders:** Containing a single constituents weighing 100 mg or more.

2. **Compound powders:** Containing more than one constituents, e.g. ORS powder.

Advantages of Powders

1. Powders are suitable form of administration for insoluble salts and for substances, which would incompatible in mixture.

2. The dose can be weighed out accurately.

3. Powders well except when they contain hygroscopic solids like sodium chloride or potassium citrate.

4. They are easy to dispense even in multiple doses.

5. Inexpensive

Disadvantages of powders

1. Difficult to mask the taste of ingredients.
2. Some people find it difficult to swallow.

A compounded prescription order

Dr R K Patil
MBBS Reg. No. 52341
KEM Hospital
Mumbai
Date:

For
Mr. Jayant Bhosale
Age: 30 years Sex: Male, Weight: 62 kg
Parsee colony, Dadar, Mumbai 400041

	g or ml	
Calamine	7	5
Zinc oxide	2	5
Bentonite	1	5
Glycerine	2	5
Rose water to make	50	0

Mix and prepare a lotion
To be applied to the affected part without friction

Doctor Sign
Stamp

Label
LOTION

Lotion

FOR EXTERNAL USE ONLY

Shake well before use

Mr Jayant Bhosale Age 30 yrs

Dadar Mumbai-41

To be applied to the affected part
without friction

GSMC Laboratories

IMPORTANT PHARMACY PREPARATION

Exercise 1

Aim: Prescribe and dispense 2 doses of sodium salicylate mixture for a patient suffering from pyrexia.

Procedure

1. Calibrate the bottle for 50 ml.
2. Weight 2 gm sodium salicylate and 1 gm sodium bicarbonate.
3. Dissolve them in 2/3 of the quantity of the vehicle.
4. Transfer the solution into the calibrated mixture bottle.
5. Add the washing of mortar and pestle to make 50 ml.
6. Label the bottle and dispense with a dose slip.

Exercise 1

Name: _____

Address: _____

Reg. No: _____

Date.: _____

For: _____

Age: _____ Sex: _____ Weight: _____

Address: _____

R̥x

g or ml

_____ | _____

_____ | _____

_____ | _____

_____ | _____

Instruction to pharmacist

Direction to patient

Doctor Sign _____

Registration No. _____

Name:

Age:_____ Sex:_____ Weight:_____

Address:_____

Direction:_____

Date:_____ Sign:_____

Solution to Exercise 1

Name: Dr ABC

Address: DEF Medical College

Reg. No.: 12345

Date: Day/Month/Year

For: XYZ

Age: 30 Sex: Male Weight: 60 kg

Address: Navi Mumbai

R_X

	g or ml
Sodium salicylate	2
Sodium bicarbonate	1
Water qs	50

Instruction to pharmacist: Mix and make a solution

Direction to patient: Divide the mixture in two parts, take one such part twice daily

Doctor sign:

Registration No.: 12345

Antipyretic Mixture

Name: XYZ

Age: 30   Sex: Male   Weight: 60 kg

Address: Navi Mumbai

Direction: Divide the mixture in two parts, take one such part twice daily

Date: Day/Month/Year   Sign:

MGM Laboratory

Application: Used in pyrexias of various etiology. As an analgesic to relative headache, bodyache or muscular pain. In cases of traumatic or degenerative inflammatory disorders, e.g. osteoarthritis

Direction: One dose to be taken 2 times a day after meals.

Action of the Compounds

Sodium salicylate: It is a salicylic acid derivative. Mechanism of action: Inhibits prostaglandin synthase and decreases prostaglandins.

Other uses of salicylate:

1. It has analgesic, antipyretic and anti-inflammatory action.
2. As a kerotolytic in warts and corns (plantar and palmar)
3. In fungal infection (ringworm, athletes foot as fungicidal and kerotolytic along with benzoic acid as fungistatic)

Sodium bicarbonate: Acts as a corrective to salicylate, to prevent gastritis that may be caused by salicylate

Other uses of salicylate:

1. As a systemic antacid in metabolic acidosis.
2. For alkalinizing urine in urinary tract infection.
3. For vaginal and urethral washes (douches).
4. For forced alkaline diuresis in barbiturate poisoning.
5. As a carminative.

EXERCISE 2

Suspension

Aim: Prescribe and dispense one dose of Mist Alba.

Procedure

1. Calibrate a clean mixture bottle for 25 ml.
2. Weight 8 gm magnesium sulphate and 1 gm of light magnesium carbonate.
3. Dissolve the magnesium sulphate in 2/3 rd of the vehicle in a measuring cylinder.
4. Prepare a uniform paste of magnesium carbonate using a part of the above magnesium sulphate solution in a mortar.
5. Transfer to a calibrated bottle after diluting it with more of magnesium sulphate solution.
6. Add the washing of mortar and pestle to make 25 ml.
7. Label the bottle and dispense with a dose slip.

EXERCISE: 2

Name: _____

Address: _____

Reg. No.: _____

Date.: _____

For: _____

Age: _____ Sex: _____ Weight: _____

Address: _____

R̥X

g or ml

Instruction to pharmacist
_____

Direction to patient
_____

_____

Doctor Sign _____

Registration No. _____

Name: _____

Age: _____ Sex: _____ Weight: _____

Address: _____

Direction: _____

Date: _____ Sign: _____

Solution to Exercise 2

Name: Dr ABC

Address: DEF Medical College

Reg. No.: 12345

Date: Day/Month/Year

For: XYZ

Age: 25, Sex: Male, Weight: 65 kg

Address: Navi Mumbai

	g or ml
Magnesium sulphate	8
Light magnesium carbonate	1
Peppermint water	25

Instruction to pharmacist: Mix and make a suspension

Direction to patient: Whole quantity to be taken in the morning before breakfast with a glass of water

Doctor sign:

Registration No.: 12345

Mist Alba suspension

Name: XYZ

Age: 25   **Sex:** Male   **Weight:** 65 kg

Address: Navi Mumbai

Direction: Whole quantity to be taken in the morning before breakfast with a glass of water

Date: Day/Month/Year   **Sign:**

MGM Laboratory

Application: Saline purgative which leads to formation of semisolid or watery stools within 2 to 3 hours.

Direction: Whole quantity to be taken early in the morning before breakfast with a glass of water.

Action of Compounds

Magnesium sulphate: Saline purgative acting on entire intestinal length. It causes release of CCK (cholecystokinin) from small intestine thus enhancing gastrointestinal motility. Given early in the morning as a single dose (draught).

Other uses of magnesium sulphate

1. Antacid by oral route along with aluminium hydroxide.
2. Orally after anthelmintic therapy or prior to the radiological examination of abdomen.
3. Systemically in treatment of eclampsia and hypertensive encephalopathy.
4. Rectally to reduce intracranial tension.
5. Topically for boils and carbuncles due to its hydroscopic action, relieves oedema.

Light magnesium carbonate: It acts as an adjuvant, potentiating the action of magnesium sulphate.

Other uses of light magnesium carbonate

1. As an antacid.
2. As a laxative.

EXERCISE 3

Emulsion (Oil/Water)

Aim: Prescribe and dispense one dose of a mineral oil laxative (O/W emulsion) in a palatable form.

Procedure

1. Calibrate a clean mixture bottle for 25 ml.
2. Weight 2 gm of gum acacia and prepare a mucilage by adding twice the amount of aqueous vehicle to the gum in a mortar.
3. Measure 8 ml of liquid paraffin in a drymeasure and add drop the contents of the mortar while trituration, until a primary emulsion is formed (indicated by the cracking sound).
4. Add more of water (continuous phase) gradually to the primary emulsion with constant trituration.
5. Transfer the emulsion to the calibrated bottle and add the washing to make 25 ml.
6. Label the bottle and dispense.

EXERCISE 3

Name: _____

Address: _____

Reg. No.: _____

Date.: _____

For: _____

Age: _____ Sex: _____ Weight: _____

Address: _____

℞

g or ml

_____

_____

_____

Instruction to pharmacist

Direction to patient

_____

_____

Doctor Sign _____

Registration No. _____

Name:

Age:_____ Sex:_____ Weight:_____

Address:_____

Direction:_____

Date:_____ Sign:_____

Solution to Exercise 3

Name: Dr ABC

Address: DEF Medical College

Reg. No.: 12345

Date: Day/Month/Year

For: XYZ

Age: 35, Sex: Male, Weight: 55 kg

Address: Navi Mumbai

R̶x

	g or ml
Liquide paraffin	8
Gum acacia	2
Water qs	25

Instruction to pharmacist: Mix and make an emulsion

Direction to patient: Whole quantity to be taken at bedtime

Doctor sign:

Registration No.: 12345

Mineral Oil Laxative Emulsion

Name: XYZ

Age: 35   **Sex:** Male   **Weight:** 55 kg

Address: Navi Mumbai

Direction: Whole quantity to be taken at bedtime

Date: Day/Month/Year   **Sign:**

MGM Laboratory

Application: This emulsion is used as emollient purgative (stool softner) in case of chronic constipation, during pregnancy, old age, in cases of anorectal problem, etc.

Direction: Whole quantity to be taken at bedtime.

Action of Compounds

Liquid paraffin: It is a hydrocarbon. It retains water by osmosis. It acts as emollient purgative making faecal mass soft. It is a mineral oil laxative.

The disadvantages of liquid paraffin are:

1. Can cause lipoid pneumonia (aspiration pneumonia) in bedridden patients.
2. Malabsorption of fat soluble vitamins on chronic administration.
3. Decreases the tone of the anal sphincter causing seeping of medicaments, staining of clothes and social embarrassment.
4. Can causes granulomas in the submucosa of the intestinal wall.

Other uses of liquid paraffin

1. Skin emollient use in dermatological conditions such as senile dry skin, dry eczema, ichthyosis, neurodermatitis, scrotal priritus and pruritus ani where it may be combined with urea and propylene glycol.
2. As lubricant for catheters.
3. Nasal lubricant.

Salient feature:

1. Takes 6 hours to act
2. Always given at bedtime
3. Avoided in ambulatory patients

Gum acacia: Source is the Acacia tree (Indian rubber tree or babul). It is an emulsifying agent.

Other stool softeners: Dioctyl sodium sulfosuccinate, sodium picosulfate

EXERCISE 4

Liniment (Oil/Water Emulsion)

Aim: Prescribe and dispense 25 ml of Turpentine liniment (O/W emulsion)

Procedure

1. Calibrate a clean mixture bottle for 25 ml.
2. Measure 16.25 ml of turpentine in a dry measure and dissolve 1.25 g of camphor in it.
3. Weigh 2.25 g of soft soap and make a solution.
4. Add the turpentine and camphor solution drop by drop to the solution of soft soap triturating continuously, till a primary emulsion is formed.
5. Transfer it to the calibrated bottle after diluting with more of water.
6. Add the washing of mortar and pestle make 25 ml.
7. Label the bottle and dispense.

EXERCISE 4

Name: _____

Address: _____

Reg. No.: _____

Date.: _____

For: _____

Age: _____ Sex: _____ Weight: _____

Address: _____

R̸x

g or ml

Instruction to pharmacist

_____

Direction to patient

_____

_____

Doctor Sign _____

Registration No. _____

Name:

Age: _____ Sex: _____ Weight: _____

Address: _____

Direction: _____

Date: _____ Sign: _____

Solution to Exercise 4

Name: Dr ABC

Address: DEF Medical College

Reg. No.: 12345

Date: Day/Month/Year

For: XYZ

Age: 22, Sex: Female, Weight: 50 kg

Address: Navi Mumbai

	g or ml	
Turpentine oil	16	25
Camphor	1	25
Soft soap	2	25
Water	15	

Instruction to pharmacist: Mix and make a emulsion

Direction to patient: Apply on affected part twice daily with rubbing

Doctor sign:

Registration No.: 12345

Turpentine Liniment

Name: XYZ

Age: 22   **Sex:** Female   **Weight:** 55 kg

Address: Navi Mumbai

Direction: Apply on affected part twice daily with rubbing

Date: Day/Month/Year   **Sign:**

MGM Laboratory

Application: Liniment turpentine acts externally in patients suffering from arthralgia, myalgia, fibrositis, lumbago, sprains, ligament tear and spin. In all these conditions it acts by the mechanism of counter irritation.

Direction: Apply on affected part twice daily with rubbing.

Action of Ingredients

Turpentine: It is a counter irritant. It is volatile oil obtained from Pinus.

Other uses of turpentine

1. To remove maggots from infected wounds.

Camphor: It is derived from wood of *cinnamon camphorea*. It is rubefacient increasing blood to the area. Never taken internally.

Other uses of camphor

1. In fainting attacks due to its strong smell
2. In urinals
3. To allay moths in cupboards
4. In pujas

Other examples of counter irritant: Eucalyptus oil, oil of wintergreen, asafoetida, ginger, etc. oil.

Salient Features

1. Never taken internally since camphor can cause erosion of mucous membranes.
2. It is a liniment, used only for external use and rubbed on skin with friction.
3. Dispensed in amber coloured bottle (for external application as it is photosensitive).

EXERCISE 5

Lotion

Aim: Prescribe and dispense 25 ml of a lotion for a patient suffering from sunburn.

Procedure

1. Calibrate a lotion bottle for 25 ml.
2. Weight 3.75 gm of calamine, 1.25 gm of zinc oxide, 0.75 g of bentonite and 1.25 gm of glycerine.
3. Triturate all these with sufficient quantity of rose water to make a uniform paste.
4. Dilute it with more rose water and transfer to the calibrated bottle.
5. Add the washing (with rose water) to make 25 ml.
6. Label the bottle and dispense.

EXERCISE 5

Name: _____

Address: _____

Reg No: _____

Date: Day/Month/Year

For: _____

Age: _____ Sex: _____ Weight: _____

Address: _____

R̽X

g or ml

Instruction to pharmacist

_____ '_____

Direction to patient

_____ '_____

_____

Doctor Sign _____

Registration No. _____

Name:

Age:_____ Sex:_____ Weight:_____

Address:_____

Direction:_____

Date:_____ Sign:_____

Solution to Exercise 5

Name: Dr ABC

Address: DEF Medical College

Reg. No.: 12345

Date: Day/Month/Year

For: XYZ

Age: 30, Sex: Female, Weight: 50 Kg

Address: Navi Mumbai

	g or ml	
Calamine	3	75
Zinc oxide	1	25
Bentonite	0	75
Glycerine	1	25
Rose water qs	25	

Instruction to pharmacist: Mix and make a lotion

Direction to patient: Apply on affected part without friction

Doctor sign:

Registration No.: 12345

Calamine Lotion

Name: XYZ

Age: 30   **Sex:** Female   **Weight:** 50 kg

Address: Navi Mumbai

Direction: Apply on affected part without friction

Date: Day/Month/Year   **Sign:**

MGM Laboratory

Application: It has protective astringent and smoothing action and therefore it is valuable in case of sunburns, eczema, dermatitis, pruritis and mild excoriations of the skin.

Direction: Apply on affected part without friction.

Action of Compounds

Calamine: It has astringent and smoothing action. It's pink colour is due to ferric oxide impurity.

Other uses of calamine

1. Sunburn
2. Urticaria
3. Insect bite
4. Photosensitivity
5. Drug allergy
6. Dry eczema
7. Acne

Zinc oxide: It has an antiseptic, astringent, antipruritis and antiperspirant effect. It also contributes to the pink colour of calamine lotion.

Bentonite: It is an adjuvant. Natural hydrated aluminium silicate with impurities.

EXERCISE 6

Ointment

Aim: Prescribe and dispense 10 gm of salicylic acid benzoic acid ointment.

Procedure

1. Weight 0.33 gm of salicylic acid and benzoic acid each.
2. Triturate them with a portion of white soft paraffin on a tile until smooth.
3. Gradually add more soft paraffin until the total weight becomes 10 gm.
4. Dispense in a grease proof paper.
5. Label the bottle and dispense.

EXERCISE 6

Name: _____

Address: _____

Reg. No.: _____

Date: _____

For: _____

Age: _____ Sex: _____ Weight: _____

Address: _____

℞

g or ml

Instruction to pharmacist
_____

Direction to patient

_____

_____

Doctor Sign _____

Registration No. _____

Name:
Age: _____ **Sex:** _____ **Weight:** _____
Address: _____
Direction: _____
Date: _____ **Sign:** _____

Solution to Exercise 6

Name: Dr ABC

Address: DEF Medical College

Reg. No.: 12345

Date: Day/Month/Year

For: XYZ

Age: 26, Sex: Male, Weight: 54 Kg

Address: Navi Mumbai

	g or ml	
Benzoic acid	0	33
Salicylic acid	0	33
Yellow soft soap	10	

Instruction to pharmacist: Mix and make a ointment

Direction to patient: Apply twice in a day on the affected part

Doctor sign:

Registration No.: 12345

Ointment

Name: XYZ

Age: 26   **Sex:** Male   **Weight:** 54 kg

Address: Navi Mumbai

Direction: Apply twice in a day on affected part

Date: Day/Month/Year   **Sign:**

MGM Laboratory

Application: It is an antifungal ointment if the concentration of salicylic acid is more useful in treating corns and warts.

Direction: Apply twice in a day on the affected part.

Action of Compounds

Salicylic acid: Bacteriostatic, fungicidal, kerotolytic

Other uses of salicylic acid

1. Use in epidermohytosis, dandruff, psoriasis
2. 2–4% is used in talcum powder.

Benzoic acid: Antifungal and antibacterial action and use as preservative for food product (0.2%).

Soft paraffin: Ointment base.

Salient features

1. Ointment in the eye is called oculentum.
2. Ointment is generally used on non-hairy skin and lotion on hairy skin.
3. Whitfield ointment is 3% salicylic acid and 6% benzoic acid in the ratio 1:2.

EXERCISE 7

Powder

Aim: Prescribe and dispense 5 gm of ORS powder for a child suffering from mild dehydration.

Procedure

1. Weight 0.9 gm of sodium bicarbonate, 0.4 gm of potassium chloride and 5 gm of glucose powder (to be dissolved in 250 ml of boiled and cooled water).
2. Mix the salts and glucose together
3. Powder them finely in a mortar, in this compound powder of ORS the substances are mixed in ascending order of their weights with the help of powder knife/spatula on a white paper.
4. Wrap it in a paper of 10 × 7.5 cm size, apply the label on the wrapping paper and dispense.

EXERCISE 7

Name: _____

Address: _____

Reg. No.: _____

Date: _____

For: _____

Age: _____ Sex: _____ Weight: _____

Address: _____

℞

g or ml

Instruction to pharmacist	

Direction to patient

_____

_____

Doctor Sign _____

Registration No. _____

Name:

Age:_____ Sex:_____ Weight:_____

Address:_____

Direction:_____

Date:_____ Sign:_____

Solution to Exercise 7

Name: Dr ABC

Address: DEF Medical College

Reg. No.: 12345

Date: Day/Month/Year

For: XYZ

Age: 10, Sex: Female, Weight: 30 kg

Address: Navi Mumbai

R̩X

	g or ml	
Sodium bicarbonate	0	9
Potassium chloride	0	4
Glucose powder	5	
Water	250	

Instruction to pharmacist: Mix and make a powder

Direction to patient: Dissolved the contents in 250 ml of previously boiled and cooled water and give sip by sip. It should be given 8 hours before preparation.

Doctor sign:

Registration No.: 12345

ORS powder

Name: XYZ

Age: 10   Sex: Female   Weight: 30 kg

Address: Navi Mumbai

Direction: Dissolved the content in 250 ml of water and give sip by sip. It should be given 8 hours before preparation

Date: Day/Month/Year   Sign:

MGM Laboratory

Application: Symptomatic treatment of diarrhoea due to any cause in children and adults.

Direction: Dissolved the contents in 250 ml of previously boiled and cooled water. Take a glassful after every loose stool.

Action of Compounds

Glucose: It creates an osmotic gradient due to which electrolytes follow the gradient and get absorbed.

Super ORS is fortified with aminoacids.

Homemade ORS: To 1 litre of boiled and cooled water add 4 to 5 pinches of salt and 4 to 5 teaspoons of sugar (1 glass is 1 pinch of salt and 1 teaspoon sugar).

Powder Packing

1. Put the powder in the centre of the paper. The size of the paper should be 10 cms × 7.5 cms.
2. Bend near the border over until it is about 1.5 cm from the far end.
3. Turm the margin of the far end and bend over to form a flap.
4. Fold flap loosely on itself.
5. Turn both side edges on the opposite sides that are in apposition with one another.
6. Pack the folded packet in an envelope and label it on the front side.

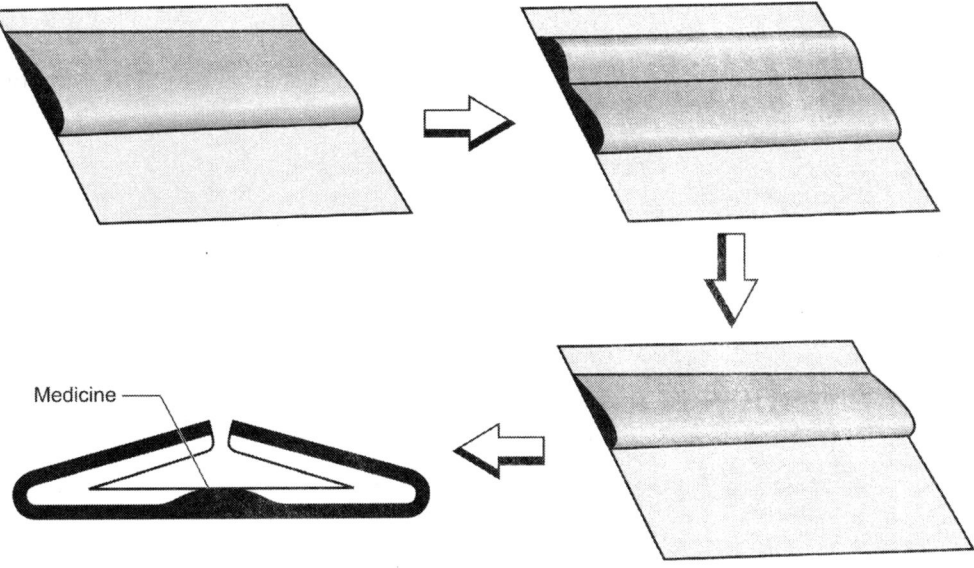

Fig. 17.1

Experimental Pharmacology

18. Introduction to Experimental Pharmacology

19. Regulations for Use of Animals for Experiments and Research

20. Animals used in Experimental Pharmacology

21. Animal Experiments

Introduction to Experimental Pharmacology

The use of animals in experimentation for the purpose of education, training and research is known as animal experimentation. The use of animals in research has resulted in the greatest drug discoveries in the 19th and 20th centuries. The first Nobel prize in 1901 in medicine was for serum therapy and research involving use of horses. Behring used horses for production of diphtheria antitoxin and the development of a vaccine against diphtheria and tetanus. The latest 2012 Nobel laureates in physiology or medicine also worked on animals. Thus, a strong association exists between rapid progress in experimental pharmacology and progress in clinical medicine.

Drug Discoveries that Involved Use of Animals

Year	Discovery	Animals used	Scientists
1901	Diphtheria tetanus antitoxin	Horses	Adolf Von Behring
1922	Insulin	Dogs	Frederick, Banting, Macleod
1939	Prontosil: 1st drug for bacterial infections	Mice	Gerhard Domagk
1941	Penicillin	Rats	Alexander Fleming
1952	Streptomycin	Chicken	Waksman

Primary Uses of Animals in Experimentation

In India, Animals are Used in Pharmacology for the following

Education

- **Undergraduate teaching:** To demonstrate the effects of drugs on various systems. Typical experiments included effect of various drugs on bioassay of guinea pig ileum, rabbit intestine, rabbit eye, screening of central nervous system drugs, frog heart and frog rectus. The latter have however declined owing to the ban on use of frogs. However, most medical colleges have begun using or in transition phase to implement alternatives to animal experiments in undergraduate course such as CAL based animal experimentation software

- **Postgraduate teaching:** To demonstrate the effects of various drugs, to determine the nature of an unknown drug for bioassay, screening methods and to learn skills, e.g. administering drugs. Toxicity studies, animal models for various disease conditions and short procedures (oral feeding parenteral injections, blood collection techniques) are an integral part of postgraduate training. The syllabus of MD pharmacology, has animal experiments as one of the major components.

Research

- Animals have been used and are still permitted for screening for drugs, in bioassay and for preclinical testing including general and specific toxicity studies. This preclinical safety and efficacy data is needed for submission to drug regulatory authorities before the permission for further studies in humans are granted.
- A larger number and a greater variety of animals are used in pure research than in applied research. This usually involves studies on embryogenesis, developmental biology, behavior and breeding in fruit flies, nematodes, mice and rats.
- Applied research that aims to answer specific questions is usually carried out in the pharmaceutical industry or by universities. Animal models of disease, discovered or generated by pure research programs, are used for applied research. Examples include use of transgenic animals, animal models of naturally occurring diseases, induced animal models of human diseases, cosmetic testing and toxicity studies.
- Rodents (rats, mice) and non-rodents (rabbits) are usually preferred for studies.

Regulations for Use of Animals for Experiments and Research

The CPCSEA provides guidelines for performing experiments on animals and maintenance of animal house. The registration of animal house is mandatory with CPCSEA and is to be renewed every 3–5 years. Besides the rules and procedures laid down by the CPCSEA, the Indian National Science academy (INSA) and Indian Council of Medical Research, have also formulated certain guidelines for care and use of animals in scientific research as well as in medical colleges.

Animals Used in Experimental Pharmacology

1. Rat (Adult Weight: 200–250 gm): It is a warm blooded rodent. It can't vomit and does not possess the vomiting center. It has no tonsil and gallbladder in its body.

Biological name: *Rattus norvegicus*

Common strain used: Albino rats of Wistar strain, Sprague-Dawley, Wistar Kyoto.

Uses in Experimental Pharmacology

- Psychopharmacological studies.
- Study of analgesics and anticonvulsants.
- Bioassay of various hormones such as insulin, oxytocin, vasopressin, etc.
- Study of estrus cycle, mating behaviour and lactation.
- Studies on isolated tissue preparations like uterus, stomach, vas deferens, anoccoccygeus muscle, fundus strip, aortic strip, heart rate, etc.
- Chronic study on blood pressure.
- Gastric acid secretion studies.

2. Guinea PIG (Adult weight: 400–600 gm): It is a docile animal. It is susceptible to tuberculosis and anaphylaxis. It is highly sensitive to histamine and penicillin.

Biological name: *Cavia procellus*

Use in Experimental Pharmacology

- Evaluation of bronchodilators.
- Anaphylactic and immunological studies.
- Study of histamine and antihistamines.
- Bioassay of digitalis.
- Evaluation of local anesthetics.
- Hearing experiments because of sensitive cochlea.
- Study in isolated tissue specially, ileum, tracheal chain, vas deferens, teania coli, hearts, etc.
- Study of tuberculosis and ascorbic acid metabolism

3. Mouse (Adult weight: 20–25 gm): It is most widely used animal in different toxicity studies. It is a warm blooded rodent.

Biological name: *Mus musculus*

Common strain used: Laca, balb-c and Swiss albino

Uses in Experimental Pharmacology

- Bioassay of insulin.
- Toxicological and teratogenic study.
- Screening of analgesic and anticonvulsants.
- Screening of chemo therapeutic agents.
- Study related to genetic and cancer research.
- Study of drugs acting on central nervous system.

4. Rabbit (adult weight 1.5–3 kg): It is a docile animal with large ears. Usually New Zealand white rabbits are used. Rabbit is a warm blooded mammalian animal.

Biological name: *Oryctolaguscuniculus*

Strains used: New Zealand white, Himalayan black

Uses in Experimental Pharmacology

- Pyrogen testing.
- Bioassay of antidiabetics and sex hormones.
- Irritancy tests.
- Study of drug used in glaucoma.
- Screening of agents affecting capillary permeability.
- Pharmacokinetics studies.

5. Frog: (adult weight 50–100 gm): Frog is a cold blooded amphibian.

Biological source: *Rana tigrina*

Common strain used: Rana esculenta, Rana pipiens and Rana temporaria.

Uses in Experimental Pharmacology

- Study of isolated tissue like rectus, abdominis muscle, heart, sciatic nerve preparation, etc.
- To study the effect of drug acting on central nervous system, neuromuscular junction and heart.
- Whole frog is also used in screening of certain drugs like anesthetics.

Animal Experiments

The Effects of Various Drugs on Rabbit's Eye

Various drugs acting on rabbit's eye are classified under the following headings:

1. **Test drug 1:** Pilocarpine eye drops 2% (parasympathomimetic)
2. **Test drug 2:** Physostigmine eye drops 0.25% (parasympathomimetic)
3. **Test drug 3:** Atropine sulphate eye drops 1% (parasympatholytic)
4. **Test drug 4:** Phenylephrine hydrochloride eye drops 10% (sympathomimetic)
5. **Test drug 5:** Timolol maleate eye drops 0.5% (sympatholytic)
6. **Test drug 6:** Lidocaine topical solution 4% (local anaesthetic)

Aim of the experiment: To observe the changes in pupil size, light reflex, corneal reflex and Intraocular pressure (IOP) changes in rabbit's eye before and after the instillation of pilocarpine eye drops.

Procedure

The procedure followed to demonstrate the effects of various drugs on the rabbit eye are as follows:

- Restrain the animal in a rabbit holder
- Wait for 15–20 min to allow the animal to acclimatize before starting the experiment.
- Use separate rabbits for testing different drugs, unless the intent is to show potentiation or reversal of the effect of a drug administered earlier. In each rabbit, designate one eye as the test eye and the other eye as control.
- Measure the baseline pupil diameter using the pupilometer.
- Measure the IOP using the tonometer, if required.
- Test the light reflex by bringing the light beam from the torch in a rapid and smooth swing from one side onto the eye.
- Test the corneal reflex by touching the cornea near the sclerocorneal junction from one side using the cotton wool wick.
- Instil the drug to be tested in one eye (2 drops), and normal saline as control in the other eye. The rabbit eye sac can accommodate a volume of about 50 µl.
- Allow at least 30 min for the drug action to develop. The control is not expected to produce any results.
- Note any changes on inspection (e.g. conjunctival congestion and lacrimation).

- Measure the pupil diameter (whether constricted or dilated) and, if required, the IOP (whether raised or lowered) again.
- Test the light reflex (whether normal, sluggish or lost) and corneal reflex (present or lost) again.

Ideally the experiment is to be performed in an environment that is not brightly lit. Different animals should be used for testing different drugs with saline control in each experiment. Asepsis should be maintained throughout. The drug solutions should not be used if they are outdated, obviously contaminated or contain particulate matter.

Table 21.1: Shows the effect of various drugs on rabbit eye

Animal 1

Test drug: Pilocarpine 2%

Test eye: Left eye	Pupil size	Light reflex	Corneal reflex	IOP	Control eye: Right eye Pupil size	Light reflex	Corneal reflex	IOP
Before drug	5 mm	Present	Present	Normal	5 mm	Present	Present	Normal
After drug	2 mm	Present (difficult to detect)	Present	Decreased	5 mm	Present	Present	No change

Animal 2

Test drug: Physostigmine (0.25%)

Before drug	5 mm	Present	Present	Normal	5 mm	Present	Present	Normal
After drug	2 mm	Present (difficult to detect)	Present	Decreased	5 mm	Present	Present	No change

Animal 3

Test drug: Atropine 1%

Before drug	5 mm	Present	Present	Normal	5 mm	Present	Present	Normal
After drug	9 mm	Absent	Present	No change	5 mm	Present	Present	No change

Animal 4

Test drug: Phenylephrine 10%

Before drug	5 mm	Present	Present	Normal	5 mm	Present	Present	Normal
After drug	8 mm	Present	Present	Increased	5 mm	Present	Present	No change

Animal 5

Test drug: Timolol 0.5%

Before drug	5 mm	Present	Present	Normal	5 mm	Present	Present	Normal
After drug	5 mm	Present	Present	Decreased	5 mm	Present	Present	No change

Animal 6

Test drug: Lidocaine topical solution 4%

Before drug	5 mm	Present	Present	Normal	5 mm	Present	Present	Normal
After drug	5 mm	Present	Absent	No change	5 mm	Present	Present	No change

Points of Discussion

1. **Effect of pilocarpine eye drops on rabbit's eye:**
   - M_3 receptors are present in the circular muscle of iris (sphincter pupillae), ciliary muscle and lacrimal gland. Contraction of circular muscle through M_3 agonistic action causes constriction of pupil size (miosis).
   - Although light reflex is present, may be difficult to detect because the pupil is already constricted.
   - Corneal reflex is not affected as the pathway of corneal reflex is intact.
   - The ciliary muscle contraction due to stimulation of M_3 receptors opens the pores of the canal of schlemn which facilitates drainage of aqueous humour and reduces intraocular pressure (IOP).

2. **Effect of physostigmine eye drops on rabbit's eye:**
   - Physostigmine is an indirect parasympathomimetic (indirect agonist of M_3 receptors) agent. The effects of the drug on the eye are similar to pilocarpine.

3. **Effect of atropine eye drops on rabbit's eye:**
   - Atropine when instilled in eye, blocks M_3 receptors present in pupillary constrictor muscle as a consequence of which there is unopposed sympathetic dilator activity due to the action of α_1 receptor on the radial muscle of the iris resulting in mydriasis. This type of mydriasis is a passive mydriasis (indirect mydriasis).
   - There is loss of light reflex because the pupillary response is abolished due to the blockade of M_3 receptors.
   - Corneal reflex is present because the pathway is intact.
   - There is rise in intraocular pressure due to falling of iris back over the canal of schlemm because of mydriasis which obstructs the drainage of aqueous humour.

4. **Effect of phenylephrine eye drops on rabbit's eye:**
   - Phenylephrine has a greater action on α_1-adrenergic receptor and causes dilation of the pupil by agonistic action on α_1-receptors of the radial pupillary dilator muscle of iris. In contrast to atropine it produces 'active mydriasis.'
   - Light reflex is present since sphincter pupillae muscles are stronger than dilator muscle. Also corneal reflex is present as neuronal pathway is intact.
   - A rise in intraocular pressure is observed after the administration of phenylephrine eye drops. This is due to release of pigments in the aqueous humor blocking the anterior chamber angle while narrowing of the angle.

5. **Effect of timolol eye drops on rabbit's eye:**
   - Timolol maleate is a non-selective β adrenergic receptor blocking agent. It has no effect on pupil size or light reflex or corneal reflex.
   - Intraocular pressure (IOP) in the eye decreases after instillation of timolol maleate eye drops. In the eye, β receptors (largely β_2 subtype) are present in the ciliary body epithelium and blood vessels. Production of aqueous seems to be activated by a β receptor-mediated cyclic AMP-PKA pathway. β blockade blunts adrenergic activation of this pathway by preventing catecholamine

stimulation of the β receptor. Also it has been reported that β blockers decrease ocular blood flow, which decreases the ultrafiltration responsible for aqueous production.

6. **Effect of lidocaine topical solution on rabbit's eye:**
   - Pupil size, light reflex and intraocular pressure are not affected. However, corneal reflex is abolished. Lidocaine, a local anaesthetic has a direct inhibitory effect on neurotransmission of the trigeminal sensory nerve which causes loss of corneal reflex.

Effect of Atropine on Rabbit Eye Using CAL Software

Aim of the Experiment: To determine the effects of given drugs on the size of the pupil, light reflex and intraocular tension of the animal eye.

Requirements: CAL Software package.

Drugs: Atropine 1%.

Procedure

- The effects of drug on rabbit eye is demonstrated by injecting drugs into the eye using CAL Software package.
- Keep one eye as test eye and another eye as control eye.
- Inject saline in control eye and atropine in test eye.
- Measure the diameter of pupil before and after injecting drug.
- Note down IOP as low, normal or high before and after injecting drug.
- Check out light reflex before and after injecting drug.
- Tabled the data as mentioned show in Table 21.1.

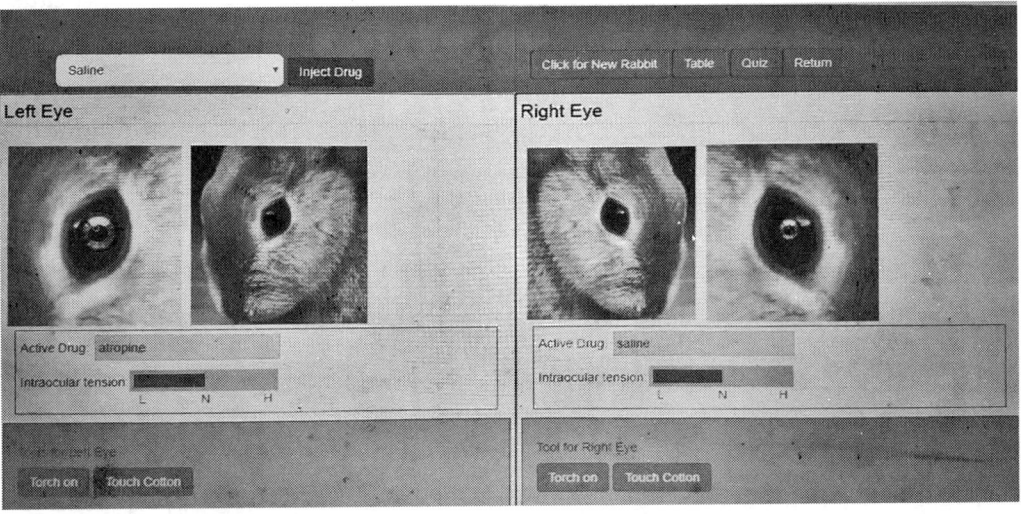

Fig. 21.1: Shows effect of atropine by using CAL software package as mentioned (left eye keet as test eye and right eye kept as control eye) (Ex-Pharm series)

Effects of Drugs on Isolated Perfused Frog Heart

Aim of the Experiment: To study the effects of drugs on isolated perfused frog heart.

Drugs tested on isolated perfused frog heart

Drugs	Dose (µg)	Concentration
Epinephrine (Adrenaline)	2	10 µg/ml
Propranolol	200	1 mg/ml
Acetylcholine	2	10 µg/ml
Atropine sulphate	20	100 µg/ml
Calcium chloride	2000	10 mg/ml
Potassium chloride	2000	10 mg/ml

Parameters to be noted

1. **Force of contraction:** Amplitude of contractile response
2. **Frequency of contraction:** Heart rate (bpm)
3. **Tone:** Determined by baseline of contractile response

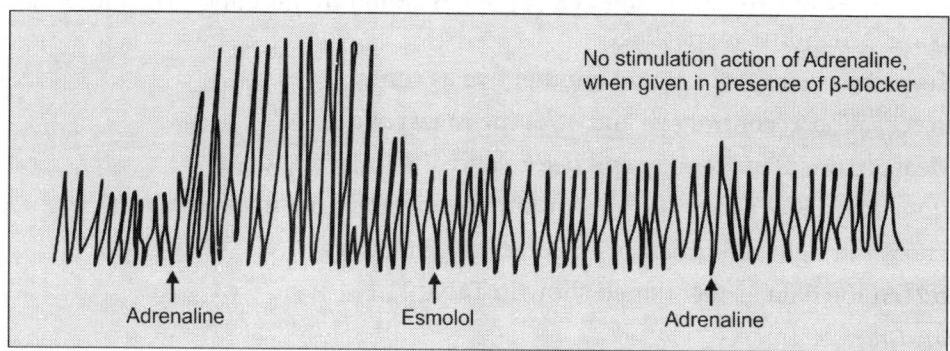

Fig. 21.2: Effect of adrenaline

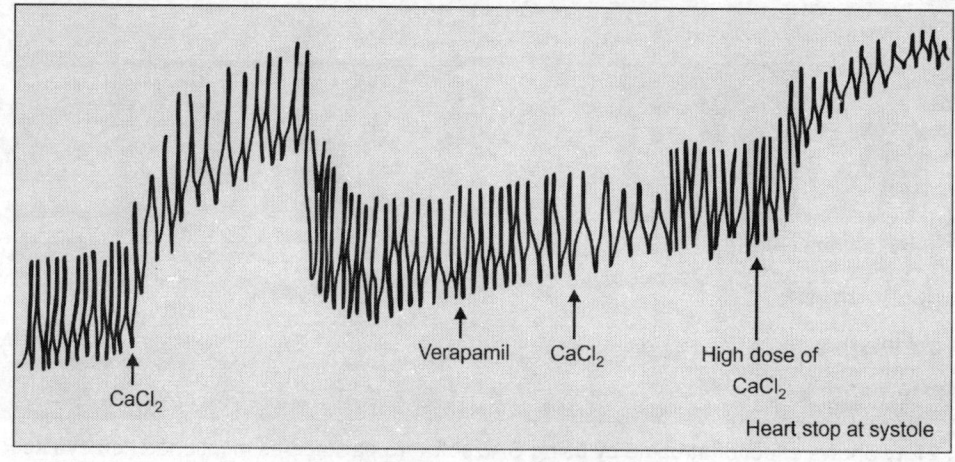

Fig. 21.3: Effect of calcium chloride

Effects of stimulant action of the drugs on isolated perfused frog heart

Test drugs which act as stimulant

1. Adrenaline
2. Calcium chloride

Table 21.2: Effects of adrenaline/esmolol an isolated perfused frog heart

Sr. No	Drug	Effects of drug on isolated perfused frog heart	Explanation
1	Adrenaline	Amplitude: Increased Heart rate: Increased Tone: Normal	Adrenaline increases the frequency and force of contraction due to the action on beta adrenergic receptors of heart. It has no effect on tone of cardiac muscle
2	Esmolol	Amplitude: Normal Heart rate: Normal Tone: Normal	Esmolol acts as an antagonist. It blocks the beta adrenergic receptors without producing any intrinsic activity (in human heart esmolol decreases the heart rate and contractility of heart muscle which is not seen in isolated perfused frog heart since the central nervous system is damaged and the heart is functioning on its own.
3	Esmolol followed by Adrenaline	Amplitude: Normal Heart rate: Normal Tone: Normal	Beta blocker blocks the β_1-receptors of the isolated perfused frog heart and antagonizes the action of adrenaline. Therefore the stimulatory action of adrenaline is blocked.

Table 21.3: Effects of calcium chloride/verapamil on isolated perfused frog heart

Sr No	Drug	Effects of drug on isolated perfused frog heart	Explanation
1	Calcium chloride	Tone: Increased	Calcium chloride is a directly acting stimulant. It increases the force of contraction but with incomplete relaxation. The tone of cardiac muscle is increased and the baseline of contraction is shifted upwards (step ladder pattern of contraction is observed).
2	Verapamil followed by calcium chloride	Amplitude: Normal Heart rate: Normal	Verapamil is an L-type calcium channel blocker. The stimulatory action of calcium chloride in presence of verapamil is blocked.
3	High dose of calcium chloride	Tone: Increased	High dose of calcium chloride causes persistent systole leading to cardiac arrest, i.e. heart stops at systole. An upward shift in the baseline of contraction is observed.

Effects of Depressant Action of the Drugs on Isolated Perfused Frog Heart

Test drugs which act as depressant:

1. Acetylcholine
2. Potassium chloride

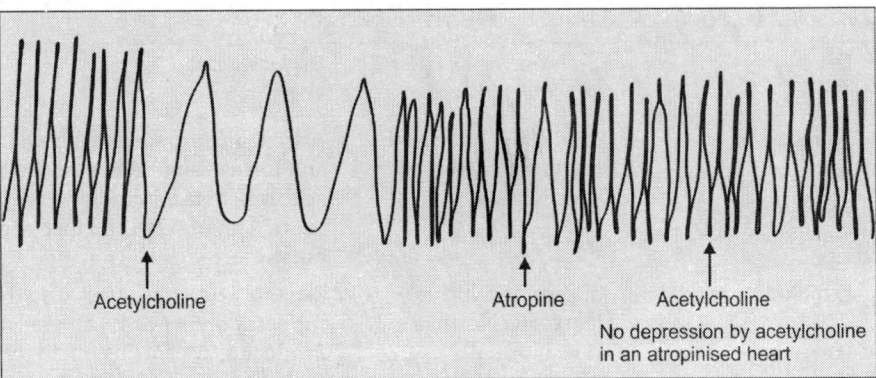

Fig. 21.4: Effect of acetylcholine

Table 21.4: Effect of acetylcholine/atropine on isolated perfused frog heart

Sr No	Drug	Effects of drug on isolated perfused frog heart	Explanation
1	Acetylcholine	Amplitude: Decreased Heart rate: Decreased Tone: Normal	Acetylcholine is a parasympathomimetic drug. It acts on the muscarinic (M_2) receptors of the heart and decreases the amplitude and frequency of contraction.
2	Atropine	Amplitude: Normal Heart rate: Normal Tone: Normal	Atropine is a parasympatholytic drug. It blocks the muscarinic receptors of the heart and produces no significant effect on contractility and heart rate because it is an antagonist and lacks intrinsic activity.
3	Atropine followed by acetylcholine	Amplitude: Normal Heart rate: Normal Tone: Normal	Atropine is a parasympatholytic drug. It blocks the muscarinic receptors and antagonises the action of acetylcholine. Therefore, depressant effect on the heart is not observed.

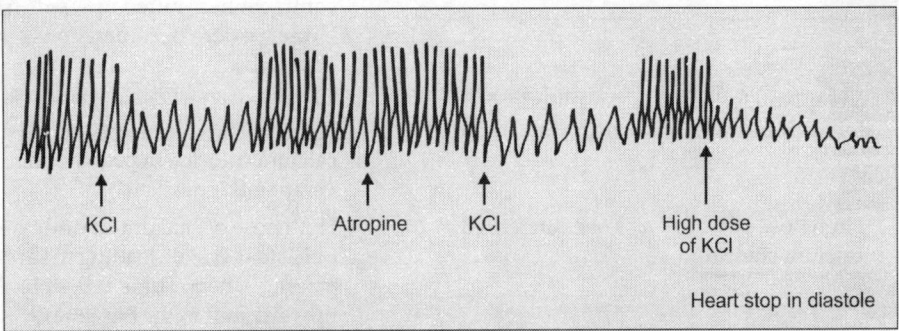

Fig. 21.5: Effects of potassium chloride

Table 21.5: Effect of KCL/atropine on isolated perfused frog heart

Sr No	Drug	Effects of drug on isolated perfused frog heart	Explanation
1	Potassium chloride (KCL)	Amplitude: Decreased Heart rate: Decreased Tone: Decreased	Potassium chloride is a directly acting depressant of the cardiac muscle, thus decreasing force, frequency and tone of contraction.
2	Atropine followed by potassium chloride (KCl)	Amplitude: Decreased Heart rate: Decreased Tone: Decreased	Atropine fails to block the depressant action of KCl since KCl is a directly acting depressant.
3	Potassium chloride in high doses	Amplitude: Decreased Heart rate: Decreased Tone: Decreased	Due to persistent depressant action of potassium chloride on heart, the heart stops at diastole.

Effects of Drug on the Isolated frog Heart Using CAL Software Package

Aim of the experiment: To study the effects of calcium chloride on the isolated frog Heart
Requirements: CAL software package
Drugs: Calcium chloride 2000 ug

Procedure

- Inject drug using CAL software package
- Observe following parameters like heart rate, amplitude and tone
- Tabulate the data as follows:

Drug	Heart rate/min	Amplitude	Tone
Control (initial reading)			
Calcium chloride			

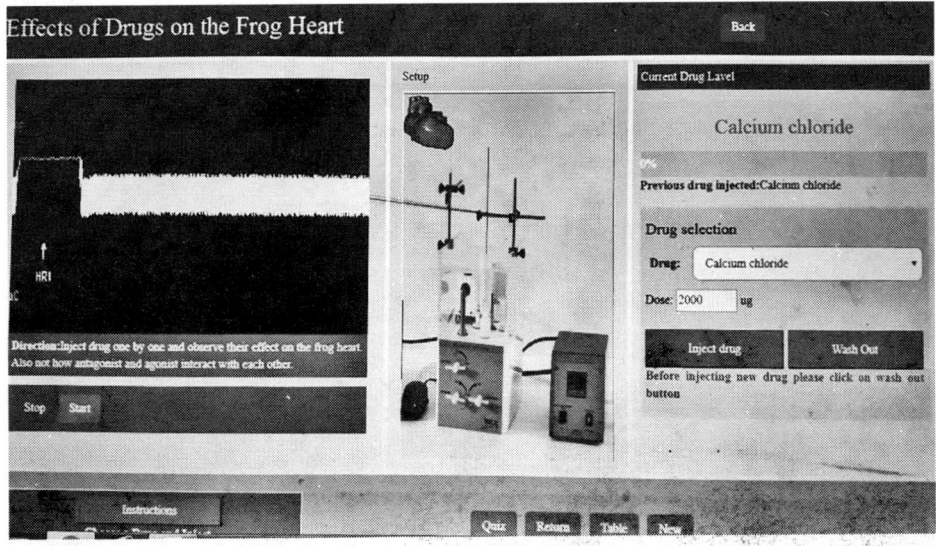

Fig. 21.6: Shows effect of drug on isolated frog heart using CAL software package

Section

D

Protocol Writing

22. Protocol Writing

23. How to Write ICMR-STS Project by Undergraduate Students

Protocol Writing

HOW TO WRITE PROTOCOL

Research Protocol

This is the document that describes the objectives, design, methodology, statistical considerations and organization of the research. The protocol usually gives the background, rationale for the research. The protocol complies by following parts:

I. Study title

II. Study summary

III. Study description:

- Background and rationale
- Objectives
- Methodology
- Data management and analysis

IV. Ethical considerations

V. References

I. Study title: Study title should be brief, specific and concise. The title should closely reflect the objective of the study.

II. Study summary: The summary of the study should include all the elements of the protocol. It should highlight the important aspects of the study in a concise manner.

III. Study description:

A. Background and rationale: Summarize and synthesize the available research (including published data) to provide justification for the study. Evaluate prior research for relevance to the research question under study. When the proposed research is the first of its type to involve human participants, the results of relevant animal studies must be included.

- Discuss the anticipated results and potential pitfalls.
- Describe the significance of the research including potential benefit for individual subjects or society at large.
- Discuss how public health and social welfare might be enhanced.

B. Objectives: Specific objectives are statements of the research question(s). The purpose of the study (research questions and/or study objectives) should be clearly and succinctly stated. The objectives are either primary that answer the major questions that the study addresses or secondary, the minor questions answered by the study. Objectives should be simple, specific, and stated in advance.

C. **Methodology:** Methods for study, data collection and for avoiding/minimizing subject risks should be included. Include a time line for subject evaluations and the duration of subject participation in the project. Identify the plans that are the proposed safeguards for subject confidentiality.

Methods will vary with the research approach used (qualitative, quantitative). The selected methods should be sufficiently described to justify the use of the approach for answering the defined research question. Methods should also be described in adequate detail.

Elaborate description as to how the study would be undertaken should be written in the methodology section. It contains the most important part of the protocol. The methodology includes information on the research design, the sample size, research subjects, interventions, observations and sample size. The following should be included in the methodology section.

– *Research design*: The research design should be identified and should be appropriate to answer the research question(s) under study. Describe the type of research proposed (e.g. experimental, correlational, survey, qualitative) and specific study design that will be used (e.g. pre-test/post-test control group design, cross-sectional design, prospective longitudinal cohort design, phase III double-blind randomized control group design).

– *Sample*: Describe the sampling approach. For experimental designs, include justification for sample size determination. Identify the procedures that will be used to recruit, screen, and follow study volunteers. Specifically define the study sample (number of subjects to be enrolled, characteristics of subjects to be included in and excluded from the research).

– *Measurement/instrumentation*: Identify the variables of interest and study endpoints (where applicable). Justify measurement techniques selected. Provide validity and reliability data for selected measures.

– *Internal validity*: Threats to internal/external validity should be considered. Describe measures that have been taken to avoid study bias.

D. **Data management and analysis:** The protocol should provide information on how the data will be managed, including data coding for computer analysis, monitoring and verification. Information should also be provided on the available computer facility. The statistical methods used for the analysis of data should be clearly outlined. Specify the analytic techniques the researcher will use to answer the study questions. Indicate the statistical procedures (e.g. specific descriptive or inferential tests) that will be used and why the procedures are appropriate. For qualitative data, specify the proposed analytic approaches.

IV. **Ethical considerations:** All types of studies involving health research require ethical permissions. Whether the research is of therapeutic or diagnostic nature, the research involving human experimentation needs to go through the ethical review process. All research protocols in the biomedical field involves human subjects must include a section addressing ethical considerations. This includes the written approval of the appropriate ethics review committee, together with a written form for informed consent. In addition, the possible ethical concerns must also be discussed.

V. **References:** Include a reference list of literature cited to support the protocol statement.

PATIENT INFORMATION SHEET AND CONSENT FORM
Patient/Participant Information Sheet

Study title: Evaluation of antidiabetic prescriptions in Type II diabetes mellitus.

What is the purpose of the present study?

Purpose of study is study of antidiabetic prescriptions and evaluation of glycemic control. Study will help doctors learn more about the Type II diabetes mellitus.

What is the study procedure?

All the diabetic patients attending the medicine outdoor department will be enrolled in the study after explaining the aim of the study. Written informed consent will be obtained from each patient. Prior approval of Institutional ethics committee, hospital superintendent and from the head of the medicine department will be obtained. Patients receiving any of the antidiabetic drugs or insulin or both will be included in the study irrespective of their gender. Anatomical therapeutic classification was used to designate each drug prescribed. The data will be collected, analyzed and appropriate statistics will be applied to obtain meaningful information.

Who will do the study?

Dr Rajesh Kumar Suman/student's name

What are the risks/discomforts of taking part in the study?

As this is study involving antidiabetic prescriptions and no direct intervention there will be no direct risk involved.

What are the possible benefits of taking part in the study?

There will be no direct benefit to you from participating in this study, this study will help doctors learn more about Type II diabetes mellitus. In the future, this information may help in the treatment of patients with diabetes.

What about confidentiality? (Regarding patient identity and also during publication of data).

Patient identity will be kept secret whole time of study and during publication patients information will not be shared with any third party except proper authorities.

Will I be paid for participating in the study?

You will not be paid for taking part in this study. However, this study will help doctors learn more about the Type II diabetes mellitus. In the future, this information may help in the treatment of patients with diabetes.

Will I have to pay for any study related investigations/procedures/ treatment?

You do not have to pay for related investigations/procedures/treatment additionally done for test other then asked in prescriptions.

What do I have to do?

Are there any lifestyle restrictions? You should tell the patient if there are any dietary restrictions. Can the patient drive, take part in sport? Can the patient continue to take their regular medication, etc.?

What is the drug or procedure that is being tested?

You should include a short description of the drug or device and give the stage of development.

What will happen to the results of the research study?

You should be able to tell the patients what will happen to the results of the research. When are the results likely to be published? Where can they obtain a copy of the published results? Will they be told which arm of the study they were in? You might add that they will not be identified in any report/publication.

Who has reviewed the study?

You may wish to give the name of the Research Ethics Committee(s) which reviewed the study (you do not however have to list the members of the committee).

Whom can I contact for further information?

You can contact principal investigator. Provide contact details for further information.

Informed Consent Form

Study title: Evaluation of antidiabetic prescriptions Type II diabetes mellitus

Principal investigator: Dr Rajesh Kumar Suman

Department: Department of pharmacology

Subject Name: (Please tick mark the applicable)

1. I confirm that I have read and understood the information sheet version _____ dated _____ for the above study and have had the opportunity to ask questions.

2. I understand that my participation is voluntary and that I am free to withdraw at any time, without giving reasons, without my medical care or legal rights being affected.

3. I understand that the sponsor of the clinical trial, others working on the sponsors' behalf, the Ethics Committee, legal and the regulatory authorities will not need my permission to look at my health records both in respect of the current study and further research that may be conducted in relation to it, even if I withdraw from the trial. I agree to this access. However, I understand that my identity will not be revealed in any information released to third parties or published.

4. I agree not to restrict the use any data or results that arise from this study provided such a use is only for scientific purpose (s)

5. I voluntarily agree to take part in the above study

Subject's Name & Signature _____

Date _____

Name & Signature of Witness (impartial witness) _____

Date _____

Name & Signature of Investigator _____

Date _____

Name & Signature of LAR (Legally acceptable representative) _____

_____   Date _____

Fig. 22.1: Informed consent form

Role of LAR in Consent Process

Consent obtained from an legally acceptable representative (LAR) in a situation where a participant is not able to give informed consent:

- Unconscious
- Minor
- Suffering from severe mental illness
- Disability

An LAR is an individual or a legal body authorized under applicable law to consent, on behalf of a prospective participant, to the individuals participation in the clinical trial.

Role of Impartial Witness in Consent Process

- If the participant or LAR is unable to read/write, then an impartial witness must sign the consent form.
- An impartial witness is a person who is independent of the trial and cannot be unduly influenced by the people involved with the trial.
- Reads the ICF and any other written information supplied to the participant.
- Usually, the patient party of the subsequent patient is taken as impartial witness.

Consenting Minors

Assent: A child's affirmative agreement to be a participant in research

Child Age 7–12: Verbal consent only

Child Age 13–18: Written assent required

AV Recording of Consent

- Vulnerable participants in clinical trials of new chemical entity or new molecular entity.
- In cases where clinical trials are conducted on anti-human immunodeficiency virus (HIV) and anti-leprosy drugs, the investigator should only obtain an audio recording of the informed consent process

CASE RECORD FORM

A document designed with protocol to record data and other information on each trial subjects. It may also be called as case report form. The CRF should be in such form and format that allows accurate input, presentation, verification, audit and inspection of the recorded data. A CRF may be in printed or electronic format.

Important tips regarding CRF

a. CRF should be designed to include all the protocol-required data.
b. CRF should be user friendly with clear instruction on completion.
c. CRF should preferable be printed.
d. The data element modules should be included on per patient visit basis to prevent the protocol noncompliance.
e. It is principal investigator's duty to design and formulate CRF. Designing of CRF and production is the first and most important step of the data management process.

CRF designing and development

a. CRF designing and development process starts either simultaneously with the protocol development or after the protocol approval.
b. The first step is to have fair understanding of the protocol and primary study endpoints.
c. Based of study endpoints, critical data fields are identified and incorporated in the form of modules.
d. Each data filed should be accompanied by the appropriate CRF filling instruction in order to avoid data queries.
e. CRF instruction are in line with data validation plan and helps in uniform data collection.
f. Once the draft CRF is designed, it is appropriate to fill the protocol required data of dummy patients just to see the applicability of data fields or possible missing data fields.
g. Extra copies of CRF page like ADR, concomitant medication, etc. should be printed to meet as required.
h. Data queries on CRF should be filed along with the respective CRF page.

Case Record Form

The example of CRF for evaluation of antidiabetic prescriptions Type II diabetes mellitus.

Tick mark or write values wherever applicable   Date: _____

OPD No		Age		Gender	M/F
Height:		Weight:		Waist circumference:	
Hip circumferences		HbA1C value (Date of estimation)		FBG/PPBG RBG:	
Duration of diabetes		Family history of diabetes	Yes/No	Currently smoking If yes, duration (Year)	Yes/No
Complication:		Treatment modality		Lipid profile	
Ocular complications		OHA duration:		TC	
Nephropathy		Insulin duration:		TG	
Neuropathy		OHA + Insulin duration:		HDL	
Foot complications		Blood pressure		LDL	
Cardiovascular complications		SBP:		Atrial fibrillation	Yes/No
Specify_____					
Any other:		DBP:		Age of onset of diabetes	

Drugs Prescribed

S. No.	Name of drug	Prescribed by		Dose	Dosage form	Frequency	Duration	Cost/ tab or Inj	Total cost
		Generic	Brand						
1.									
2.									
3.									
4.									
5.									
6.									

Other concomitant medication prescribed: ....

Fig. 22.2: Case record form (CRF)

How to Write ICMR-STS Project by Undergraduate Students

Participation in research is important in producing doctors with an understanding of evidence-based medicine. Though a mandatory part in postgraduate medical course, research has largely been invisible from the undergraduation medical course in India. very few research opportunities are available at undergraduate level. The reason behind this is lack of encouragement, lack of basic infrastructure, facilities and structured mentorship programs, no extra incentives to researchers and the long journey to get academic acclaim. Another additional aspect is of lack of writing skills for biomedical publication. Additional incentives to students as well faculty members are required to foster the research environment in India.

Some Achievements of Medical Students' Research

- Jay Mclean, a medical student working at John Hopkins University, discovered Heparin.
- Lorenzo Bellini was only 19 years when he published his discovery (1662) of the kidney tubules.
- Charles Herbert Best, a medical student contribution to medicine nearly won him a Nobel Prize.
- Paul Langarhans in 1869 discovered the Islets of Langarhans which bear his name.
- A Danish anatomist, Niel Stensen was a medical student when he discovered in 1961, the parotid duct in sheep.

ICMR-STS Fellowships

The fellowships offered by Indian Council of Medical Research (ICMR) for medical students-ICMR-STS (short term studentship) Fellowships introduces the young inquisitive mind to enter into the world of research.

Background

- The Indian Council of Medical Research initiated the short term studentship program in 1979 to promote interest and aptitude for research among medical undergraduates.
- The main objective of this program is to provide an opportunity to undergraduate medical students to familiarize themselves with research methodology.

- The value of the studentship will be Rs. 10000/- per month for 2 months' duration (Rs. 20000/- only) and is meant to be a stipend for the student.

Eligibility

- This program is only for MBBS/BDS students studying in medical/dental colleges recognized by MCI/DCI.
- The student must carry out the research in his/her own medical/dental college under the guide who is employed in the medical college as a faculty.
- Only permanent full time faculty members working in any of the Department of the medical/dental college where the student is enrolled can act as the guide.
- Only one student will be allowed to work under one guide.

Procedure to Apply

- This is a fully online program. No hard copies have to be submitted.
- The student is required to register on ICMR website in the month of mid-December and then submit the application form and proposal online by January every year which will be evaluated by ICMR.
- Guide must take overall responsibility for the conduct of the research project, preparation and submission of complete report and the required enclosures within the stipulated time period.
- The selection of the candidates for award of research studentship will be done after technical evaluation of the research plan by a panel of experts.
- The student should obtain a clearance from the Institutional Ethics Committee (IEC) if the proposal involves research on human participants and from Institutional Animal Ethics Committee (IAEC) if the work involves use of animals.
- The IEC/IAEC approval should be obtained any time between January-April before the beginning of actual research work.

General Instructions

- Students are requested to visit ICMR website (www.icmr.nic.in) and comply with instructions updated from time to time about STS program.
- Students who were unable to complete their STS project can reapply for next STS program with the same project. However, it will not be given any special preference and will be treated as a fresh/new application.
- For queries send an email at stshrd2017@gmail.com and please quote the reference ID in all your e-mail correspondence for quick reference.
- Results will be announced in April and list of selected students will be displayed on the website.
- If selected, the student is expected to complete the project in any two given months between April and September every year and submit the report before the last date of submission.
- The student will be awarded stipend and certificate only if his/her report is approved.

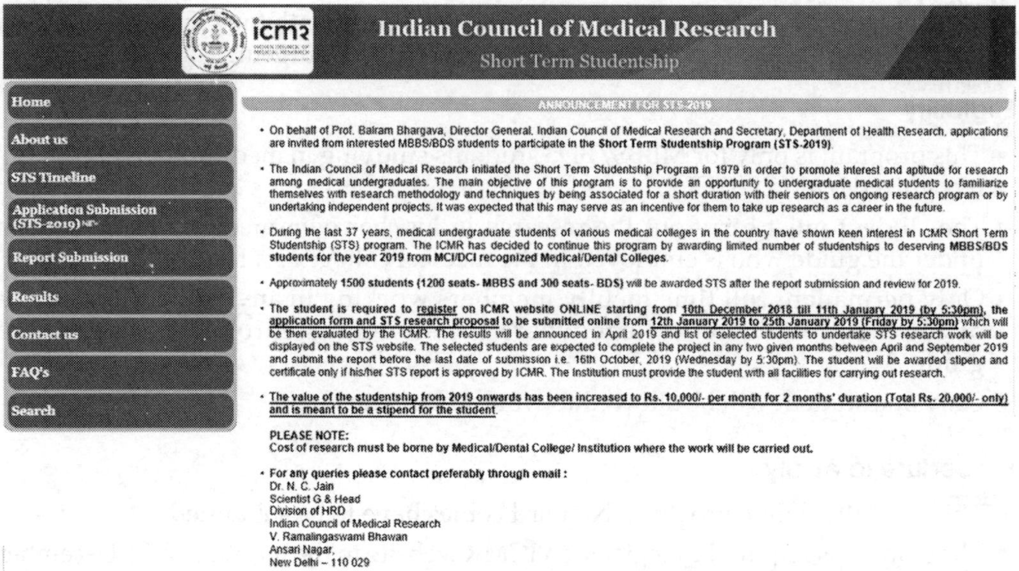

Fig. 23.1: ICMR home page

ONLINE REGISTRATION
Login and Student Course Details

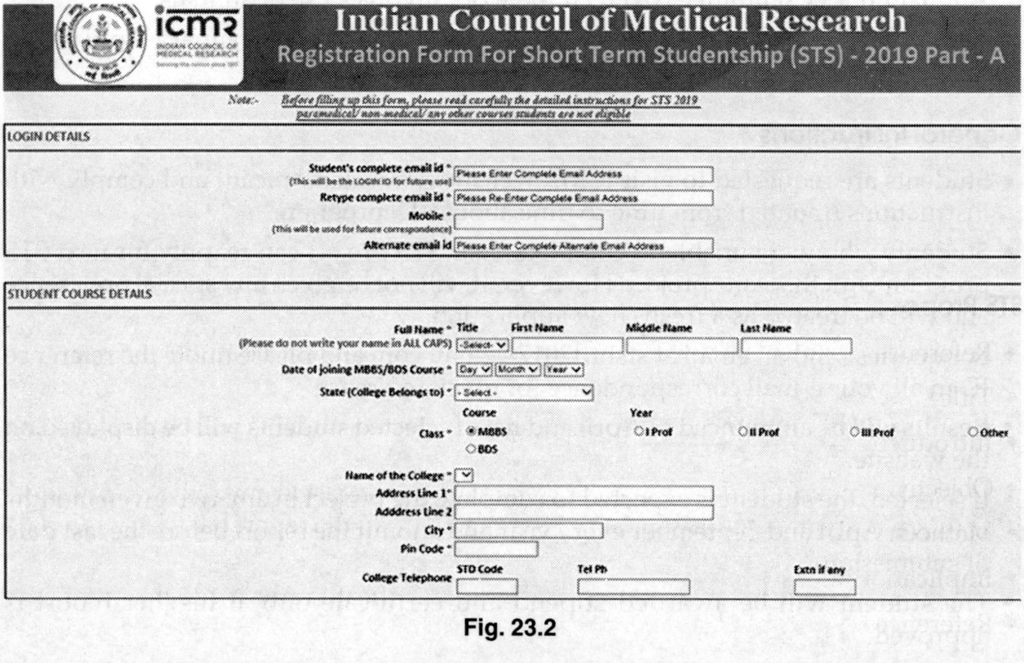

Fig. 23.2

Student Personal Details

STUDENT PERSONAL DETAILS

Gender * ○ Male   ○ Female
Nationality * [Indian ▼]

Date of Birth * [Day ▼] [Month ▼] [Year ▼]
State (Home Belongs to) * [- Select - ▼]
Home Address Line1 * [   ]
Home Address Line2 [   ]
City * [   ]
Pin Code * [   ]
Alternate Mobile [   ]

Residence Telephone STD Code [   ]   Tel Ph [   ]

Where would you want correspondence to be sent to * ○ College   ○ Home

Fig. 23.3

STS TIMELINES FOR 2019

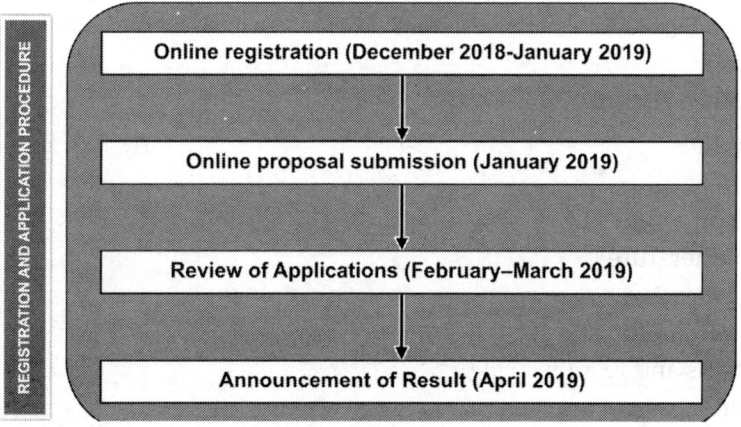

REGISTRATION AND APPLICATION PROCEDURE

Online registration (December 2018-January 2019)

Online proposal submission (January 2019)

Review of Applications (February–March 2019)

Announcement of Result (April 2019)

Fig. 23.4: Time line: Registration and application procedure

STS Proposal Details

- Reference ID   (Generated upon registration)
- Title   (25 Words)
- Introduction   (300 Words)
- Objectives   (100 Words)
- Methodology   (800 Words)
- Implications   (100 Words)
- References (Vancouver style)   (300 Words)

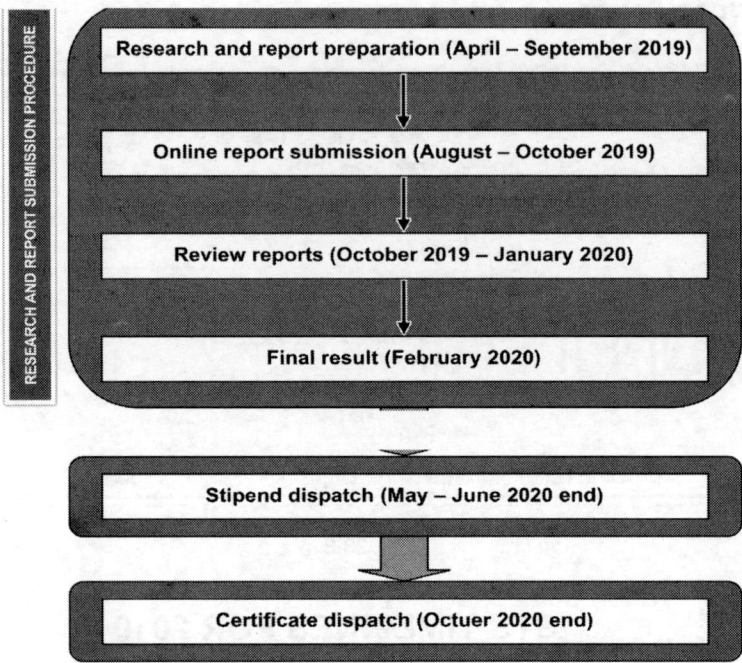

Fig. 23.5: Time line: Research and report submission procedure

STS Final Report Format

- Reference ID
- Title
- Introduction
- Review of literature
- Aims and objectives
- Material and methods
- Observations and results
- Discussion
- Conclusion
- Summary
- References

Communication Skill

24. Interaction with Pharmaceutical Representive

25. Communication with Patients

Interaction with Pharmaceutical Representative

Interaction with Pharmaceutical Representative

Physician share a very strong and unusual relationships with medical representatives. Interaction with Pharmaceutical representative is a regular phenomenon in daily life of physician.

Medical representative is essentially a catalyst who conveys knowledge on most recent trends in medical diagnostic and treatment to the physician. The interaction of pharmaceutical representative influence physician to prescribe branded costliest drug over cheap generic drug and its increases healthcare cost. The pharmaceutical industry invests heavily in promotion, and it has used a variety of promotional strategies to stimulate sales of pharmaceutical drugs. Within this context, medical representatives are the key personnel employed in promoting the products and an integral part of pharma field force. Therefore, It is important to create awareness among medical student regarding interaction with medical representative.

What doctors expect to get from medical representatives?
- An effective drug
- Information concerning the drug
- An idea concerning drug price
- Available dosage forms
- Free samples
- Brochures
- Conferences
- Services

Following are the key point that medical students should keep in mind during interaction with pharmaceutical representative
- Mentioning about international non-proprietary name
- Kindly give brief clinical information regarding the drug
- Indication of drug
- Dose range as per pharmacokinetic data
  Average dose range for adults and children
  Dosing interval
- Contraindication

- Adverse effects
- Precaution and warning
- Storage condition
- Description of the product
- Dosage forms
- Name and address of manufacturers
- Pack size of drug
- Legal category regarding drug
- Assurance to representative to prescribe their drug if it is suitable and promising
- Thank you to representative

Communication with the Patients

Health service researchers approve patient satisfaction as the key outcome indicator of medical care quality. Patient satisfaction with the physician-patient interaction indicates the level of physician's success and competence in service provision. Physician-patient communication is one of the most important parts of clinical practice. To improve doctor patient communication, it is important that physicians should follow best practices.

Use simple language: Clinical terms are used regularly in conversations between physicians, by replacing these medical terms with simpler language or preferably local language. Physicians can better inform to patients about diagnosis and treatment details, encouraging more successful outcomes.

Direct communications: Direct communications may keep patients informed and prompt more effective decision-making.

Encourage questions: Physicians can create a healthy approachable environment where patients are encouraged to ask questions. With a more open ended questions and ample time, patients can get the answers they need and take on a larger role in the decision-making process. It will help to create healthy relation between the physician and patients.

Be empathetic: Physicians visits can make a lot of patients anxious. It is important for physicians to acknowledge the patients feelings and be empathetic. This will help to improve patient's overall satisfaction.

Clear instruction: Physician can provide simple written required instructions when necessary, which will ease patient to understand better treatment details.

Make doctor patient communication meaningful: Healthy communication between physicians and patients not only can have a therapeutic effect on patients and improve their satisfaction, but it can also translate into better outcomes for their health. Incorporating the above best practices into communications may help foster a stronger physician-patient relationship. There are many barriers to good communication in the physician-patient relationship like patients' anxiety and fear, doctors' burden of work, fear of physical or verbal abuse, and unrealistic patient expectations.

Conversation between doctor and patient: When a patient approaches a doctor for sickness and gets medical assistance, the patient follows the prescription and no pharmacological instruction given by the doctor to get well soon.

Case 1: **Communication of doctor and patient where patient complaining about their stomach pain and diarrhoea**

Patient: Good Morning Doctor

Doctor: Hello! What can I do for you?

Patient: Doctor, I don't feel good.

Doctor: Softly, Tell me. What problems do you have?

Patient: I am suffering from pain in my stomach and loose motion since last night. I have also vomited a few times last night.

Doctor: What did you have yesterday?

Patient: I had some snacks on the roadside stalls.

Doctor: It is possible that you had contaminated food. Because of loose motion, you have lost plenty of body fluids. You require to be hydrated. Drink enough water regularly, at least 10-12 glasses of water. Mix Electoral powder in water and drink regularly. Avoid caffeine, dairy products and solid foods at least till evening. And get plenty of rest. I am prescribing a few medicines to control diarrhoea.

Patient: Thank you, doctor.

Doctor: you will be alright within few days, come to meet me if you get any complain. Do you have any other questions?

Patient: No, doctor. Thank you.

Case 2: **Communication during prescribing medication**

Ex: prescribing Enalapril in Hypertension

- You have been diagnosed with hypertension and treatment needs to be initiated. If left untreated it can lead to severe health complications and increase the risk of heart disease, stroke and kidney problems.
- I am prescribing you a tablet of enalapril 5 mg every day once in the morning after food.
- This drug might cause dry cough, headache, dizziness and skin rash and you need to report immediately to the physician.
- Hypertension requires long term treatment. The drug should not be discontinued abruptly as it can adversely affect your condition and might be dangerous.
- Reduce the amount of salt intake to less than 5 grams per day. Have plenty of fruits and green vegetables. Avoid consumption of processed food and sweetened beverages.

FURTHER READING

1. KD Tripathi, Essential of Medical Pharmacology (2019), 8th Edn, Jaypee Publication.
2. SK Srivastava, Pharmacology for MBBS, (2021), 2nd Edn, APC Publication.